Well Now!

Dominic Gaziano, MD

To all my patients. You inspire me every day.

To the amazing caregivers I've met throughout my career. Thank you for your commitment and often heroic efforts to care for and uplift your patients and their loved ones.

To my four brothers, three of whom took the Hippocratic Oath—Phil, Mike, Tom—and to the only brother who did not—Todd. You all helped me cultivate my critical-thinking skills as I was growing up.

To my mother and father, who taught me how to respect, empathize and communicate with others. You gave me the foundation for a life that has been truly rich and fulfilling.

Table of Contents

Part 2
Building Strong Health Care Relationships

Part 3
Being and Staying Well

Introduction

I'm Dominic Gaziano, M.D., a primary care physician who practices in inner-city Chicago. I've been in the trenches of American health care since completing my internal medicine residency, during two immensely tumultuous decades in my life. My earliest understanding of health care came from watching my father practice medicine. He was a traditionalist and I learned from his stoic ways. My father instilled in me a way of looking at life and health objectively. When I would have a minor bruise, a small abrasion, or a cold, he would say simple things like, "Wash it off with soap and water and you'll be okay," or "Wear a t-shirt when you go to bed and get some good rest and the cold will be gone." He taught me at a young age my first major tenet of self-health: don't sweat the small stuff.

Like most of you, I have witnessed profound changes in health care since my childhood. The last ten years alone have brought a dramatic shift in the economics, practice and delivery of health care in the United States. From the consolidation of medical practices—many of which are now owned by large corporations and hospital systems—to the profound changes in insurance and the cost of care, health care disruption has jeopardized the sanctity of the doctor-patient relationship.

I have watched independent medical practices disappear all around me, as doctors face mounting economic pressures. Many of them just can't hold on. Sometimes I feel like the last independent medical practice standing. Worst of all, some doctors who have moved over to a corporate environment now seem afraid to speak up when there is a clear need to change a policy or practice. In this new corporatized setting, some doctors are afraid to offend their employers. Their loss of independence on the business side has led to a loss of independence in their thinking. This shift is having a profound, negative impact on the delivery of health care in our nation.

A few groups have fared especially poorly in this transition. The poor and elderly, in particular, have seen services cut. The health care system that has evolved in the last several years doesn't serve them well. As a result, I have become a staunch defender of those who can't defend themselves—an advocate for the underdogs. My first outpatient setting after I finished my residency was at a posh downtown Chicago medical campus run by Northwestern University. Since I couldn't get excited about treating acne or allergies, I moved to Wicker Park and set up an office for low- and middle-income patients. From the moment I opened the doors, I have run my practice the way my father ran his— anyone who wants to see me can come in and see me. Giving my patients accessibility to primary health care is part of my mission. I accept all the major insurance plans, public aid and Medicare, as well as hardship patients who cannot pay at all.

Despite challenges, I am motivated to maintain an independent private practice because I believe it is the best way to serve not only the most vulnerable, but all of my patients. Staying independent allows me to keep my practice and services more affordable, efficient, direct, and compassionate. My practice is focused on the doctor-patient relationship, which I believe is central to helping my patients live healthier lives. Being the head of my own practice allows me to work with my core beliefs intact. I have the time to show my patients the respect all human beings deserve. I can focus on active listening and the type of observation and diagnostic practices that lead to useful insights about my patients' health and well-being. I strive to build strong relationships with my patients from their very first visit, though sometimes it's the second or third visit before we find a true connection. Some of my more challenging patients might not warm up to me until the fourth or fifth visit. That's fine. I find these patients the most fulfilling to treat because they often show the most dramatic improvements in their health.

Keeping my medical practice independent hasn't been easy. I've had to work an extra two to three hours a day to keep my patient volume up while providing adequate time for each appointment. My staff is forced to deal with an ever-increasing number of forms and insurance compensation decreases and denials. As a business owner, I must comply with new regulations, government oversight and constant changes in technology. For me, it's worth all the headaches. This type of simpatico doctor-patient relationship has clear benefits for my patients, especially those who face acute or chronic health concerns. My patients continue to give me insights and help me feel fulfilled in my work as a doctor. I want you all to know what a meaningful doctor-patient relationship feels like and understand how it can benefit your health and well-being. It's why I wrote *Well Now!*

The original idea came to me after I ran an online advertisement for new patients. As a result, I started seeing an increasing number of younger patients in my practice, many of whom were in their twenties. Some of them had tried to diagnose themselves through online research. Armed with the tidbits of medical information, they came into my office with fear in their eyes. Their research had led them to become overly concerned. They were anxious they might have serious medical issues. I was usually able to put them at ease in a matter of minutes, so that we could begin to focus on their actual health conditions and wellness goals.

Through ongoing discussions, I learned that many of my patients—especially those from the millennial generation—had no idea what a health care provider's role was in their lives, or how the doctor-patient relationship was supposed to work. They didn't know that a doctor could provide holistic knowledge about the body *and* mind, guide them through the medical process, advise them about their health concerns, and be their advocate. What had gone wrong? How had this disconnect between patient and doctor occurred?

I believe the answer to that question has much to do with economic and cultural reasons I mentioned at the beginning of my introduction— health care is increasingly corporate, fractionated, and expensive. The doctor-patient relationship has suffered greatly as a result.

Well Now! is a guide to show you how to take control of your own health and health care. It's my hope that it will help bridge the chasm that has developed between doctors and patients.

How to Use this Book Effectively

The goal of this book is to equip you with the skills and tools you need to take care of yourself and advocate for yourself in a variety of situations. The information is presented in three parts:

In Part One, "Understanding You and Your Health," I explore the concept of self-health in more detail. We'll start with an assessment of your health, and I'll show you how to take an honest look at your own biases, fears, stresses and other roadblocks that can interfere with a straightforward assessment of your health and treatment options.

Part Two is called "Building Strong Health Care Relationships." Here, I will help you learn to find the right health care provider and build your health care dream team—which can include not only your doctor, but your pharmacist, produce person, psychologists, psychiatrists, healers, spiritual guides, physical therapists, chiropractors, personal trainers and even your "health buddy." It will help you understand medical jargon and show you the right way to approach your team and get the most out of every interaction you have with them. It will also demystify the health care system, and give you tips on how to navigate the murky waters of insurance and costs.

In Part Three, "Being and Staying Well," we'll look at the best sites for doing online research and sharing what you find with your doctor. We'll also look at how you can be prepared for emergencies and how to navigate emergency facilities when necessary, as well as ways you can reward yourself for achieving your health goals. We'll explore how to use vacations and staycations to reduce stress, and finally, how to pay it forward to your family and community by sharing your own story.

Feel free to jump around to chapters and topics based on your interest—we all do it. However, if you read *Well Now!* in a more methodical, beginning-to-end way, you're going to have a stronger sense of the building blocks you need to take care of yourself in a variety of health situations and a clear-cut path towards achieving a state of self-health.

PART **1**

UNDERSTANDING YOU AND YOUR HEALTH

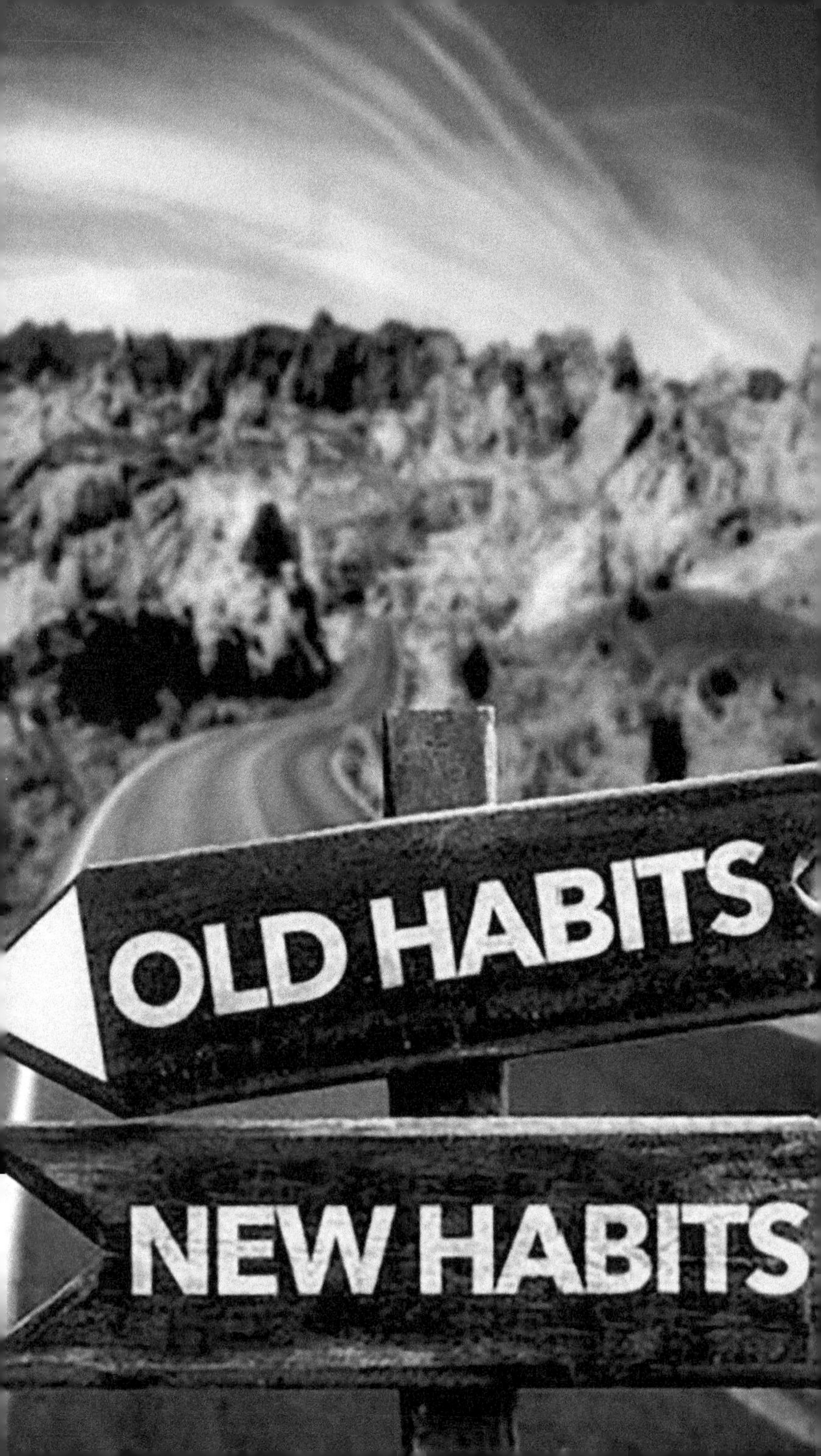
OLD HABITS
NEW HABITS

CHAPTER 1

Your Self-Health Plan

> *"A goal without a plan is just a wish."*
> *Antoine de Saint-Exupéry*

We all know individuals who always have a healthy glow and seem to waltz through life with a beautiful inner peace. How have they achieved this state of health and well-being? What's their secret? Truth is, they don't have any special knowledge that the rest of us lack. They simply follow a daily routine that makes their health a priority. They eat right, work out, relax when they can, and generally seem to make time to enjoy life. Whether they recognize it or not, they have a self-health plan that lets them reap the benefits of a life well lived.

What is Self-health?

You'll see the term self-health often in this book. So, what does this term mean? Self-health embodies the idea that *you* take complete responsibility for your health. It means you educate yourself about your body and learn to apply correct remedies for minor aches, pains and other maladies. Even better, you strive to prevent many medical issues with a proper diet, exercise, and a relaxed mental state.

Self-health is something of a movement in the medical world, a concept that emerged as a way to combat the increasing price of health care. You can easily see how preventing problems can lower costs. Treating your symptoms without entering the medical system is an important way to reduce health care costs, and also part of the self-health movement. Yet many in the medical community do not encourage the practice of self-health. They're still focused more on curing diseases rather than preventing them in the first place.

Self-health also draws on the principles of integrative medicine, which embraces many different practices, both traditional Western ones, Eastern ones such as acupuncture, and alternative treatments like massage therapy and herbal remedies.

To practice self-health you must embrace these four core principles:

- **Recognize that you are the sole person responsible for your health**
  Don't count on anyone else. Your parent, spouse, child, or friend couldn't possibly care more about your health than you do. You must take the lead. Others can give you advice, but you should be in charge.

- **Organize your schedule to achieve your health and wellness goals**
  This may seem obvious, but it's not that easy to do. Being fit and healthy takes time. We'll explore some ideas about how to do find the time you need for self-health in the next chapter.

- **Pursue current and reliable health and wellness knowledge**
  The Internet is full of information about health. But a whole lot of false information is out there, too. It's provided by everyone from pharmaceutical companies to outright witch doctors. I'll show you in another chapter how to verify that you're getting medical information you can trust.

- **Practice healthy habits every day**
  I know...this sounds like something your mother would say. It's so obvious that you're

likely to dismiss it as a no-brainer. But think about what it really means. Think about how your life could change for the better if you could replace bad habits with good habits—more energy, more focus and clarity, better health and well-being. That's huge! I'll give you strategies to practice healthier habits later in the book.

The Mind and Body Connection in Self-health

Think about it. If your body is in perfect health, strong and vibrant, but your mind is a mess—full of negative thoughts, self-doubt, anxiety and stress—you're really not well. Or...you may be happy as a lark when you sit down in front of the TV every night with a bag of potato chips and a diet soda. Your mind may be completely free of stress, financial concerns or unhappy thoughts, but if your ankles are swollen and it's painful to walk, you're not really well. Self-health means a state of wellness in *both* mind and body.

The mind-body connection has been accepted by health practitioners for centuries, and now has been conclusively proven by many scientific studies. It's clear that people in good emotional health are better able to pay attention to their thoughts, behaviors, and moods. Your psychological state has to be in good working order to lay a foundation for physical wellness. So now let's tie this mind-body connection back to you. To practice self-health you must be able to:

Manage your stress

Too much stress puts a strain on both mental and physical health, causing weight gain, poor memory, and insomnia, among other symptoms. At best, these symptoms interfere with optimal health. At worst, they make can make you ill and cause disease. In fact, this can become a vicious, self-perpetuating cycle. Stress and anxieties sneak up on us in subtle ways. If we don't identify and proactively address problems, they can eat away at your sense of well-being and cause damage.

Control your weight

As a doctor who regularly treats the negative health consequences of being overweight, I've learned to talk frankly about the importance of weight control in order to help my patients understand what they should weigh and help them develop a plan to achieve meaningful weight loss, if weight is an issue.

Eat right

Unfortunately, in general, the medical community doesn't focus like it should on proper nutrition. A basic understanding of nutrition is very important if you want to maintain a self-health plan as well as prevent other medical conditions, like diabetes and high blood pressure. Just because your weight is in the correct range for your age and height, don't assume you're getting all the nutrients your body needs to perform optimally. That's not always the case.

Stay fit

According to the Center for Disease Control, 80% of American adults are not getting enough exercise. Are you one of those Americans? If so, it's time to turn to the "Fitness Trio"—cardio, resistance, and flexibility exercises. They are all very important to achieving optimal wellness and for keeping you looking and feeling healthy. Staying fit is necessary for self-health.

Practice integrative health

Integrative medicine focuses on care of the whole person—body, mind and spirit. It combines a wide range of therapeutic approaches by a variety of health care practitioners—both from Western research-based and holistic practices. It's a team approach that helps patients achieve optimal health and wellness in all areas of their life. Integrative medicine focuses on prevention, rather than disease treatment.

Stress and Self-health

Through the years, I've gotten a tremendous satisfaction from being able to comfort my patients and help them deal with their stress. Patients have shared a variety of their stressors with me—everything from the complications of urban living (even having a loved one murdered), to breakups, divorces, job losses, and battling major diseases. It makes me feel like a true healer when I can help get them back up on their feet.

When I sit down with my patients, I direct the conversation to at least eight major causes of stress: health concerns, work-related problems, financial challenges, relationship trials, media overload, environmental factors, poor nutrition, and insufficient sleep. I bet most of the stresses in your life fall under these categories.

My experience treating patients has brought me to the conclusion that any stress can be conquered. There are many well-known stress management techniques you can use to develop your coping skills. They include yoga, meditation, relaxation tanks, hypnosis and biofeedback.

One method I like to use is a stress diary. Carve out a few minutes in your day to vent. Write down everything that is stressing you out—without questioning its validity. Minimizing the scope of your issues only conceals them and hinders you from confronting them. After you've had a break, maybe a cup of tea or a brisk walk, come back with a problem-solving mindset and have a fresh look at what your list of stresses shows. Maybe they happen at a certain time of day. They might be related to a specific person or a particular combination of circumstances. Look for ways you can minimize or reduce the stresses.

As you learn to practice self-health, you'll begin to change your mind-set in many ways. Dealing proactively with stress will become a priority—something you plan. The downtime required to relax and escape life's stressors will become a necessity, not a luxury. You'll begin to replace old patterns of dealing with stress—comfort-eating or drinking too much, for example—with new, healthier patterns like exercise or having a warm cup of decaf tea or glass of milk before bed.

Sleep for stress management

Adequate sleep is critical for stress management. Sleep times vary depending on your age and individual needs, but seven to nine hours a night are recommended for most adults. If you are constantly sleep-deprived, you are at greater risk for weight gain, heart disease, poor performance, and even diabetes. For optimal health and well-being, try to establish a consistent sleep and wake routine built around the same times every day (or at the very least on work days).

Stretching before sleep can relax your muscles. Slow, mindful breathing, meditation and dark or softly lit rooms can help you fall asleep faster. Clean and comfy clothing, along with setting the thermostat to a cool but comfortable 65 degrees, allows your body to regulate itself in a way that doesn't keep you awake. Getting the right amount of sleep will empower you in your health journey and give you the energy you need to exercise, make healthy choices, and ultimately live a fulfilling life.

Arianna Huffington has written a book about the importance of sleep and different ways of getting your sleep hygiene in tune with your self-health objectives. You can find twelve tips from her at http://ariannahuffington.com/sleep-resources.

Exercise for stress management

Once you have identified your major life stressors, consider exercise to alleviate your stress symptoms. Your body produces natural painkillers called endorphins that are released with exercise, and they can greatly reduce stress. Have you ever heard of athletes who run long distances and get what is called a "runner's high"? Well, this state of euphoria is caused by the release of those natural neurochemicals into the brain. Endorphins can elevate your mood to a level during (or after) your workouts that will have you wondering what you were so worried about in the first place. These powerful neurochemicals will put you in a more relaxed, mellow state.

The benefits of exercise extend beyond the release of endorphins. There are social and emotional rewards as well. For example, if you work out with a group, you can benefit from being around positive, energetic people on a regular basis. At first, exercise might seem like a "chore." Over time, though, you're likely to look forward to your workouts, even if just for the company of the friends that you've made. The workout will become an escape—one that is much healthier than smoking cigarettes or drinking heavily to get away from the day's stress.

The American Heart Association recommends that you get 150 minutes of moderate exercise or 75 minutes of vigorous exercise each week. This roughly equates to four, 40-minute sessions of moderate exercise a week or three, 25-minute sessions of vigorous exercise each week. It's a good idea to start slow and work your way up to more vigorous exercise.

When you become physically fit, emotional fitness comes hand-in-hand. As you begin to see positive physical results from your workouts, you will start to feel more confident and relaxed. You will sleep better too.

Relaxation techniques for stress management

Breathing techniques can relieve stress by quieting the mind and relaxing you quickly wherever you are—at work, school or home. To begin, find a quiet place and quiet part of your day when you will not be interrupted. If you do a Google search for "breathing exercises," you'll find links to all kinds of techniques for centering yourself by paying attention to your breath. There are instructions for alternate nostril breathing, deep abdominal breathing, and many more approaches. There's even an animation with a circle that expands when you are to breathe in, and contracts when you are to breathe out. You quickly fall into the peaceful rhythm. Yoga classes are also a good way to pay attention to your breathing.

Many people like to meditate. They find it brings them an inner calmness. There are many types of meditation from transcendental to heart rhythm, kundalini, guided visualization, qi gong, zazen and mindfulness. Some are upward meditation, some are downward. Upward means the exercise is drawing energy upwards and consciousness out of the body. Downward is when you invite energy down into your body through your heart. Do a Google search for "meditation techniques" and you'll be presented with a fascinating menu of different ways to explore this stress-reducing experience.

Weight and Self-health

Weight is many people's biggest health issue—no pun intended. To manage your weight, you first have to determine what your ideal weight should be. Your ideal weight will depend on your desired BMI (Body Mass Index), body fat, your age, and other factors. BMI is calculated using your height and weight and assigns a number value to your size. Find a reliable BMI calculator such as the one on the National Heart, Blood, and Lung Institute's website. (www.nhlbi.nih.gov). Ideally your BMI should fall somewhere between 18.5-24.9. Values above or below this specified range can indicate that you are under or overweight. (http://www. calculator.net/ideal-weight-calculator)

There are cases where the BMI can be misleading. Athletes with higher muscle density will weigh more and can thus be considered overweight. The elderly who lose muscle mass with age may end up with readings that wrongly classify them as underweight. This is why you should calculate your body fat percentage along with your BMI just to be sure. You can determine this value by using calipers to pinch at your skinfolds or measuring tape with an appropriate body fat calculator like the one on the American Council on Exercise's website (www. acefitness.org). A body fat percentage above 32% for women and 25% for men is considered obese. A body fat percentage in the lowest categories, along with a BMI under the normal range, can indicate being underweight. However, a similar body fat percentage paired with an "overweight" BMI reading can indicate a muscular body.

There are various approaches to weight management. Assessing your daily calorie intake is a great place to start. Calorie counters can help you gauge just how many calories you can eat to maintain or increase your current weight, and what your limit should be if you want to lose weight. The American Cancer Society has a calculator on their website (https://www.cancer.org/healthy/ eat-healthy-get-active/take-control-your-weight/ calorie-counter-calculator.html). An app like MyFitnessPal provides a richer user experience, complete with fields to record what you eat and how long you exercise each day. It also has a database of nutrition facts.

If, on the other hand, you need to gain weight, you will need to find ways to consume extra calories, especially if you burn a lot of calories through physical activity. You'll need to increase your meal portions and consume foods that are calorie dense. You might consider eating more than four meals spaced throughout the day.

Some people have metabolic disorders, which the Mayo Clinic defines as a cluster of conditions including increased blood pressure, high blood sugar, excess body fat around the waist, and abnormal cholesterol or triglyceride levels that occur together, increasing your risk of heart disease, stroke and diabetes. These are serious medical conditions, that diet and exercise alone might not address. They include things like an especially large waist circumference, or extremely high blood sugar, increased thirst or urination, fatigue and blurred vision. If you suspect a problem, you should see a doctor to determine the cause.

As we've discussed before, practicing self-health requires a certain mindset and a plan. It means taking control of your life and making your health a scheduled priority in your day. With regard to weight loss, this comes down to meal planning. Stocking your pantry with the foods you need to achieve your optimal weight requires organization. You'll need to research recipes and healthy snacks, make a grocery list to find the proper ingredients, make time for regular visits to the grocery store, prepare meals and snacks in advance, so you can grab them when needed during your busy work week.

One of the easiest things to do to lose a lot of pounds in the beginning is to simply stop eating out. In Spring 2017, *Time* magazine looked at a study that examined 150 overweight individuals who had to check in every day to report the temptations and cravings they were having. What they found out is that these individuals had less of a desire to overeat when they were at home, and that places like restaurants and bars brought about the most temptation when it came to unhealthy foods and drinks.

People often forget to reward themselves after they have reached a certain weight goal. Rewards are important because they keep you motivated, and they are an incentive that can actually make you look forward to your exercise that day. But, this reward doesn't have to be in the form of food. For example, if you drop ten pounds in certain amount of time, take yourself out to movie or buy yourself a new outfit. You deserve it.

Nutrition and Self-health

The Centers for Disease Control reports that American adults aren't eating enough fruit or vegetables. Most are only eating fruit once a day, and vegetables a bit less than twice a day. Overall, women were found to consume more produce than men, and young adults consumed fewer fruits and vegetables than all other age groups.

Dietary guidelines from the U.S. Department of Agriculture recommend at least two-and-a-half cups of vegetables, and two cups of fruit per day. That's anywhere from five to twelve total servings of fruits and vegetables. If we presume that one cup of fruit or vegetables is equal to one serving, this means that most of us are missing out on quite a bit of essential nutrients and antioxidants, all of which are necessary for maintaining good health and preventing disease.

So, how can you incorporate more fruit and vegetables into our diets? What does the optimally nutritious shopping cart and grocery list look like? You start by creating your optimal nutrition plan. Government websites such as MedlinePlus (www.medlineplus.gov) and ChooseMyPlate (www.choosemyplate.gov) provide information that can help you examine foods and put together healthy meal plans. It is important to get yourself on the right track by eating a varied diet that includes all of the necessary food groups. They'll also give you information on the three macronutrients you should be tracking. These are carbohydrates, fats, and proteins. Each of these macronutrients play a different role in your body's health, and each are vitally important.

Carbohydrates

Sometimes, people talk about going on a low-carb diet, and instead of counting calories, they'll count carbs. Carbohydrates are essential to your body's overall well-being; they fuel your body during high-intensity workouts, are its main source of fuel during digestion, and help in weight-management by making you feel fuller longer. They may even help prevent cardiovascular disease. For these reasons, it's important to include the right amount of sugars, fiber, and starch in your diet. The Mayo Clinic recommends that no more than 45 to 65 percent of your daily caloric intake should be carbohydrates. So, if you're on the standard 2,000-calorie diet, this means you'd get about 900-1,300 calories from sugars, starches, or fiber per day.

Although carbohydrates are essential for your health, not all carbohydrates are created equal. Foods such as fruits and vegetables are rich in fiber and should make up more of your daily caloric intake than foods containing a lot of added sugar, like cookies and candy. Whole grains like brown rice and whole wheat bread should always take priority over refined grain products, such as white bread and pasta.

Protein

Functioning as one of the building blocks of the body, protein is another macronutrient that is essential to your optimal nutrition plan. Formed by long chains of smaller units called amino acids, protein builds the tissue structure of your skin, hair, nails, muscles, bone, blood plasma, and organs. Your metabolism, hormones, and your body's delicate balance all require protein to function properly. Some proteins contain too much fat—think red meat or bacon—and others lack the full complement of nine amino acids the body needs to digest them properly. On a standard 2,000-calorie diet, you should be getting 10 to 25 percent of your daily calories from protein-rich foods such as seafood, meat, poultry, eggs, nuts, seeds, legumes, and soy.

Fat

Over the years, fat has gotten a particularly bad rap as the number one cause of heart disease and other ailments. More recently, however, scientists have uncovered the essential role "good fats" play. Good fats—like polyunsaturated omega-3 fatty acids—serve as a fuel reserve, protects vital organs, insulate your body, and transport fat-soluble vitamins such as vitamin A and E.

While fats are essential to your overall well-being—just like carbohydrates and protein— not all fats are good for you. The American Heart Association recommends that you incorporate poly- and mono-unsaturated fats into your diet for optimal health but limit your consumption of saturated fat due to its potential to cause heart disease. Poly-unsaturated fats can be found in sunflower seeds, almonds, and soy beans. Mono-unsaturated fats can be found in olive oil, peanut butter, avocados, and most nuts and seeds. Saturated fats on the other hand come mainly from animal sources, usually meat and dairy products. Fatty beef, lamb, pork, butter, cheese and whole or 2% milk are some examples. You should only eat these things in moderation—or not at all.

By doing the right research you can figure out what foods you should put into your shopping cart. It's important to make a grocery list so you don't forget anything crucial to a new recipe. Choose lean proteins, some whole grains, and plenty of vegetables. Limit your intakes of saturated fats, sugars, salts, and alcohol. When you get to the grocery store, take the time to read labels and choose lower calorie options. Nutrition Facts labels will give you percentages of fats, carbohydrates, fiber, sodium, cholesterol, and other vitamins and minerals. Stay away from the center aisles of the store, which are typically laden with prepackaged foods loaded with added sugars and refined carbohydrates. Be sure to pick up some healthy snacks as well, such as protein bars with less sugar, wholesome crackers, bags of nuts or dried fruits. That way you won't be tempted to turn to a candy bar at 4:00 in the afternoon.

As you approach the checkout line, your cart should be full of leafy greens like spinach or kale, fruits such as bananas and apples, red and orange vegetables like tomatoes or carrots, and whole grains like brown rice or quinoa. Occasionally, it's okay to indulge in a little ice cream or other treat. Just be sure to read the nutrition label and be mindful of your portion size.

Deciphering the Nutrition Facts Panel

The Nutrition Facts panel is there for a reason: to help you make healthy choices about the food you eat. Always start with the serving size. On virtually all nutrition panels, you will find the number of servings per package as well as the serving size, or the amount you should have per sitting. The amount per serving will usually be listed in cups and then followed by grams. All caloric values and nutritional information on the top part of the panel are for an individual serving of the product.

Next, the panel tells you how many servings of the food there are in the package. For example, if a box of elbow macaroni has two servings per box, with each serving being one cup, then consuming the entire box means consuming twice the number

Nutrition Facts

Serving Size 2 Rounded Scoops (
Serving per Container 20

Amount Per Serving

Calories 150   Calories from Fat 40

% Daily Value*

Total Fat 3.5g	**5**%
Saturated Fat 0g	**0**%
Trans Fat 0g	
Cholesterol 0mg	**0**%
Sodium 180mg	**8**%
Potassium 60mg	**2**%
Total Carbohydrate 15g	**4**%
Dietary Fiber 5g	**20**%
Sugars 1g	
Sugar Alcohol 5g	
Protein 21g	**42**%

of calories listed on the panel. In other words, to find out how many calories you've just consumed, you'd have to double all values found on the label.

Take a look at the sections labeled "Calories" and "Calories from Fat". A calorie is an efficient measurement of how much energy the food provides for your body. Unfortunately, most people consume more calories than their body needs, which leads to weight gain. Using this section, you can control your portion sizes and thereby control your caloric intake. For example, if you ate a pint, or two cups, of 200-calorie ice cream every night before bed, you're eating 400 total calories in all. In order to find out just how much fat you're ingesting, you can look at the "Calories from Fat" section. If the ice cream above had 100 calories from fat, then you'd be eating 200 calories from fat each night. Further down on the label, you will find the list of nutrients per serving. First, the label lists the nutrients you should limit in your diet. These values tell you the total fat, saturated fat, sodium, and cholesterol per serving. After those values, you'll find the values for good things like dietary fiber, vitamin A, vitamin C, iron, and calcium. In general, many Americans are not eating adequate amounts of these vitamins. Not getting enough calcium puts you at risk for developing osteoporosis. Last but not least, the note at the bottom of the panel tells you the values for the standard 2,000 or 2,500-calorie diet. Using this information, you can determine how much calcium, for example, the cup of yogurt you'll be having for breakfast provides.

Fitness and Self-health

Self-health is about way more than calorie intake. It's also about exercise and fitness—which is the way you burn calories. Building more lean muscle through exercise will increase your sitting or resting metabolism. This, in turn, will help you burn even more calories and increase your overall energy level. Daily exercise sets up a virtuous cycle in your self-health journey. You feel more vital and have a more positive outlook toward your health and weight loss. You improve your chances of losing weight because you're burning more calories, even when you're not exercising. You have better mental clarity and focus. Working out becomes something you look forward to each day, rather than a chore. Start your new fitness program slowly. You may feel soreness during the first few weeks, but that's okay, the soreness will soon go away. Work your way up to where you can combine all three types of exercise listed below.

Cardio

Cardio is any exercise that raises your heart rate. It's also often referred to as endurance or aerobic exercise. Hydration before, during and after exercising is an especially important factor with cardio, so be sure to drink plenty of water.

Cardio can be either low- or high-intensity, depending on what you do and the speed in which you do it. You could walk, jog, run, sprint, ride a bike, or even dance. Cardio is extra important for your heart and lungs; it really gets your blood pumping and maximizes your airflow. Start by choosing a good low-intensity exercise to warm up, like walking or jogging. If you are already pretty physically active, this should be a breeze. If you don't have any major heart problems, you can go ahead and add in periodic sprints to really get your heart pumping. High-intensity intervals like short sprints are an excellent way to get your heart rate up quickly. A five-minute intense interval is enough time to get your heart going strong, but not so long that you get physically exerted.

If you don't want to commit yourself to—or can't afford the expense of—a gym membership, you can establish a dedicated workout area in your home by purchasing as little as an exercise mat, a pair of weights, and a jump rope. If you don't have the time for a full 20- to 30-minute workout, find ways to sneak in physical activity throughout the day. This might consist of running up and down the stairs instead of taking the elevator, parking further away from work and power-walking to the office, planking, or doing squats while watching TV. For maximum effectiveness, the shorter the workout, the more intense it should be.

Resistance

Resistance training consists of various different exercises that force your skeletal muscles to contract, resulting in increased muscle mass, strength and tone.

The most common forms of resistance exercises use your own body weight such as with push-ups, pull-ups and squats. Others include weights and stretch bands, which can be either on machines or just individual weights and bands.

Start with just your body weight and try some push-ups and squats. Work on your form and practice. Try a few things before you jump right into something that might be too much for you. It is best to figure out what you are comfortable with and capable of doing and then work your way up to other things. Try to find exercises that work multiple muscles for the most efficient results. It is wise to take a couple breaks and do some light stretching to keep your muscles' mobility at their best. After doing a few different exercises for somewhere around ten minutes, then gently stretch those same muscles that you just used for a minute. Continue that cycle again with other muscle groups.

Flexibility

Flexibility is your range of mobility. As you age, your flexibility can start to decrease, especially if you are inactive. The benefits of flexibility training include reduced risk of injury, improved posture, greater freedom of movement, reduced muscle tension and soreness, and physical and mental relaxation. Flexibility can be improved by stretching. Studies are now proving stretching is best after or even during work outs instead of before like previously thought. But the training does not have to be just stretching; other activities can be a flexibility exercise. A good example is slowly running in place or walking briskly for a few minutes.

At the end of your resistance or weight-lifting session, you should always spend at least five minutes stretching your tightened muscles. If your personal trainer mentions you need to focus on flexibility with longer sessions, you might try a type of yoga or Pilates where you're stretching for the full session. Avoid stretching too far; do only as much as is comfortable, and then feel the muscles stretch just barely past that—enough that it slightly increases your range of motion but does not hurt you.

Balance is an important element in your exercise routine. As you will see, balance is involved with most physical activities and we use it a lot without even realizing it. An absolutely perfect way to include balance into your routine is by practicing yoga. Yoga can be for all ages and all health levels. You can start out easy, doing only as much as you are comfortable with, and work your way up to more challenging positions. You will get better the more you do it, and you'll feel great too. It is also extremely relaxing and a good way to wind down after exercise.

Integrative Health Maintenance for Self-health

Integrative health maintenance is a proactive approach that goes beyond preventing and curing disease. In addition to reducing potential health complications, the goal of integrative health maintenance is to help the person become more in tune with his or her body, mind and spirit. Armed with the knowledge imparted by a diverse team of health and wellness advisors, anyone can achieve optimal health and wellness. It is an approach that can greatly improve the overall quality of a person's life.

The medicine I practice intentionally combines the best of research-based holistic medicine with research-based Western medicine. My years at the University of Cincinnati and Northwestern University gave me the foundation I needed to practice Western medicine. Fortunately, I had the opportunity to head up the integrative medicine program at a hospital in Chicago, where I learned a great deal from various brilliant holistic practitioners—chiropractors and practitioners of Reiki and Qi Gong, for example. It changed my understanding and practice of medicine because I saw it work time after time. The thirty-year-old patient whose shoulder pain from being on the computer all day kept him hunched over was able to stand up straight after a Shiatsu massage. An eighty-year-old woman who experienced severe pain in her elbow walked out of an acupuncture session totally pain free. Soon I came to believe that tearing down the walls between various approaches to medicine and integrating everything that works—for whatever reason—was the best way to heal people.

In a self-health plan, being open to integrative health is key. I'll give you an example that illustrates the continuum of integrative medicine. Say you have a mild asthma attack. I'd recommend first trying a cup of herbal tea to counteract it. It's a natural bronchodialator and will open up your airways. But if you progress to a moderate or severe attack, go see your Western-trained MD.

In conclusion, none of us is ever going to escape the random medical problem: a broken bone, high cholesterol, an unexplainable skin rash. But if you approach your aches and pains with the support of a robust self-health plan you'll be better able to make good decisions and save money by treating what you can yourself, and knowing when to see a doc.

Dr. G's Takeaways

- Self-health requires you to embrace four core principles: recognize that you are the sole person responsible for your health; organize your schedule to achieve your health and wellness goals; pursue current and reliable health and wellness knowledge; and practice healthy habits every day.
- It is important to identify stressors in all areas of your life in order to overcome the unhealthy symptoms they create.
- Adopt relaxation, meditation and breathing techniques to combat stress.
- Regular exercise and good nutrition are vital to maintain health.
- Take your weight control and fitness goals seriously and plan for success by scheduling the time you need to organize and shop for healthy foods as well as exercise.
- Practice integrative health by getting age-appropriate screenings and discussing a holistic prevention plan with your doctor.
- Make a plan for self-health and stick to it. You'll reap the rewards for the rest of your life.

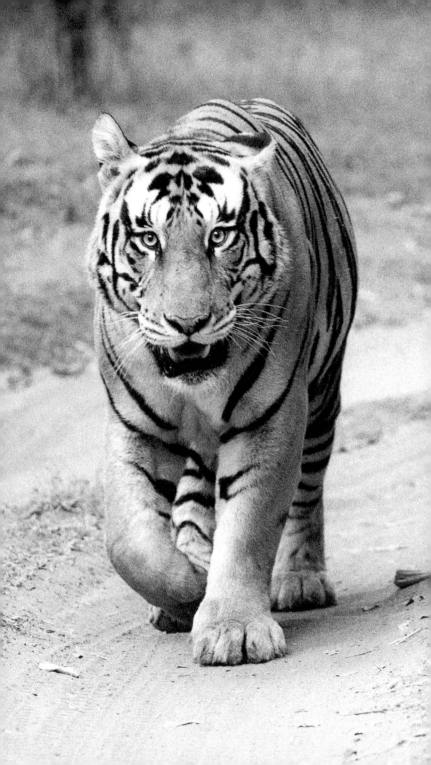

CHAPTER 2

Roadblocks to Self-health

> "A further sign of health is that we don't become undone by fear and trembling, but we take it as a message that it's time to stop struggling."
>
> Pema Chödrön, *The Places that Scare You*

Most people desire to be healthier. If you've decided it's time to establish a self-health plan, you'll need to learn the habits and practices required to be healthier as well as the challenges and roadblocks that can prevent us from reaching our self-health goals. Let's start by taking a look at those mental and emotional roadblocks that hold us back. What I see the most in my practice is patients who struggle with fear, stress and loneliness. These are significant forces in their lives that prevent them from achieving optimal health and well-being. And, let's face it, it's difficult to change and easy to make excuses when you're trying to embrace significant lifestyle changes while juggling the many competing priorities of your busy week. We're going to take a look at some of the most common excuses, and how to tackle them, so you can achieve your self-health goals.

Fear as a Roadblock

One of the primary roadblocks to good health is fear. Think about it. You put off going to the doctor because you're afraid you'll discover bad news. Maybe you avoid stepping on a scale because you're afraid it will show that you put on ten pounds in the last month. Perhaps you're afraid of the pain or embarrassment posed by a particular medical procedure you need.

We all have fears about different aspects of our lives. These fears act as a roadblock to achieving our self-health and other goals. Suppose you're walking along a country road and there is a tiger in the middle of the road staring at you. Your options are to go forward and face the tiger, choose an alternate route and attempt to go around the tiger, or turn around and go back to where you started. (At any time, you can also call Animal Control who can humanely deal with this dangerous situation.) In life and in health, we are often faced with dangerous "tigers"—fears we have created in our minds that prevent us from being happy and healthy.

Let me give a health-related example. You're in the critical second week of trying to lose twenty pounds. You step on the scale and, to your vast dismay, discover that you haven't lost any weight. The fear tiger appears and blocks your road to weight loss, saying, "You will never succeed in losing this weight. You can't do it. It's not possible...not for you!" The sad thing is *you* created that fear tiger. Maybe the very first time you tried to lose weight after high school, you failed. Multiple times in the past several years you tried to lose weight and again failed. Each failed attempt reinforced your belief that weight loss is not possible for you. In essence, you'd been going to the zoo for many years, feeding the fear tiger ever since it was a cub and watching it grow.

Perhaps the fear tiger has unexpectedly shown up at other times in your life. You didn't get that promotion, so obviously you aren't worthy of being promoted. You didn't meet your financial goal for the year, so you never will. The fear tiger that you let loose is affecting many aspects of your life and now the fear tiger is big with peering eyes. It's standing in the middle of the road staring you down every time you want to go somewhere. Then, one day, the doctor says you're overweight and it's affecting your blood pressure. This puts you at a much higher risk of a heart attack. Suddenly, you have no choice but to face the tiger. And you can. You can tame the tiger and put it right back in its cage at the zoo. You just need to breathe, research the problem, and reach out to your doctor. Think of your health care provider as your animal control person. They can help you understand and treat the problem that is causing you to be afraid and help you address it head on. They have the knowledge and tools to help you put that tiger back in its cage.

Stress as a Roadblock

We all have varying degrees of stress in our lives. For some, stress is manageable. For others, stress becomes a roadblock for developing important daily habits to become healthier. The trouble starts when we feel we can't work through our stress. We become anxious, disorganized, or unable to focus on anything positive. The key is to be able to develop coping mechanisms and become more resilient...to become hardy. By definition, the word hardy means capable of withstanding adverse conditions. Hardy people look at problems differently. They tackle problems head on and bounce back quickly. The goal of stress management is to become hardier.

You have to have a certain mindset to become hardy. You have to think about the things that stress you out as problems to be solved, rather than life stressors to be tolerated. Think about an epic hero like Indiana Jones. He's faced with life-threatening scenarios in almost every scene of his movies. It would be a very short film if he just let the giant boulder roll over him or the warriors chasing him actually kill him. Instead, he studies the problem and overcomes it. And every time he finishes confronting one obstacle, he gets back up to confront the next one. Indiana Jones is a very hardy guy! Think about the daily obstacles in your life—perhaps they are related to your health, finances, relationships, or something else. You don't have to be Indiana Jones to shift your mindset and start thinking of life's daily obstacles as just one more problem to be solved. You just need a hardy mindset, some information to help you assess the situation and a plan to overcome the obstacle. If you can address stress in this way, you can tackle anything life throws at you. If you struggle with stress in your life, developing a hardy approach to life should be an important self-health goal.

Loneliness as a Roadblock

National Public Radio recently covered the topic of loneliness in a May 1, 2018 in a piece entitled,

"Americans Are A Lonely Lot, And Young People Bear the Heaviest Burden." Here's what they reported:

Loneliness isn't just a fleeting feeling, leaving us sad for a few hours to a few days. Research in recent years suggests that for many people, loneliness is more like a chronic ache, affecting their daily lives and sense of well-being.

Now a nationwide survey by the health insurer Cigna underscores that. It finds that loneliness is widespread in America, with nearly 50 percent of respondents reporting that they feel alone or left out always or sometimes.

Using one of the best-known tools for measuring loneliness — the UCLA Loneliness Scale — Cigna surveyed 20,000 adults online across the country. The University of California, Los Angeles tool uses a series of statements and a formula to calculate a loneliness score based on responses. Scores on the UCLA scale range from 20 to 80. People scoring 43 and above were considered lonely in the Cigna survey, with a higher score suggesting a greater level of loneliness and social isolation.

More than half of survey respondents — 54 percent — said they always or sometimes feel that no one knows them well. Fifty-six percent reported they sometimes or always felt like the people around them "are not necessarily *with* them.» And 2 in 5 felt like «they lack companionship,» that their «relationships aren›t meaningful» and that they «are isolated from others.»

The survey found that the average loneliness score in America is 44, which suggests that "most Americans are considered lonely," according to the report released Tuesday by the health insurer.

It's clear that loneliness is on the rise in America. Many cultural, technological, economic and societal shifts have contributed to this unsettling development. As a nation, we're going to have to figure out what's going on and make some changes. For me, however, I try to tackle lone-liness one patient at a time. Every month in my practice, I see more patients who are getting sick because they are lonely.

Because I work hard to understand both the physical and emotional needs of my patients, I can often tell when loneliness is contributing to a patient's declining health and well-being. Some of these patients don't live alone, but they are lonely nonetheless. My lonely patients are often gripped by obsessive thinking and illogical fears about their health. They may show early signs of depression through a tendency to slower move-ment and speech patterns. Many harbor anxiety and suffer from general anxiety disorder. They complain about somatic body conditions such as abdominal or chest pain. I am not alone in see-ing the correlation between loneliness and health. There is a growing body of reliable research that correlates loneliness with illnesses such as depres-sion, social anxiety, addiction, sleep disorders, and other health conditions.

When you are lonely, emotional support is the most important type of support you can receive. Don't be afraid to ask for help. You don't have to do everything on your own. Do not isolate your-self from your support base, thinking they won't understand. When I was in college I worked for a cancer information hotline to help counsel patients with cancer. The oncologist who was the head of the program told all the volunteers that the number one fear of cancer patients is not death, but abandonment. I have taken this to heart my entire medical career, and whenever I have to tell a patient bad news, I remind them that they have a great team, and I explain specifically how my team is going to help them deal with their diagnosis.

My Personal Journey Through Stress, Loneliness and Depression

I can empathize with my patients who are dealing with stress, loneliness and depression because I have walked in their shoes. Three different times in my life, I let stress get the best of me. I didn't know what I know now about the dangerous consequences of too much stress, undeveloped coping mechanisms and isolation. Here is my story.

During my second-year of medical school, I was not doing well. My grades were not where I wanted them to be. I was struggling academically. Though I had been social in high school, college, and medical school, I gave it all up and isolated myself in order to turn things around. I spent hours in the stacks at the library, keeping myself in a corner to study. As my isolation and stress increased, my emotional health declined. I went down, way down. I believe I was clinically depressed.

As I reflect back on it now, the people who performed best in medical school were the ones who stayed connected to their family and friends. Those who had regular contact with their support network were the most successful. I, on the other hand, had lost my connections and it made me dysfunctional. I knew I had to change and change quick. I started to participate in some of the study groups that had formed at my school. A woman in my class named Rachel saw that I was struggling and made a point to draw me out a bit. I got through this difficult time with her support, and I learned a crucial life lesson.

Unfortunately, my journey with depression was not over. When I moved to Chicago after medical school, there was a lot of change in my life. I had broken up with my girlfriend, rented a new apartment in a new city, and was starting a new job. I was also preparing for my board exams, and once again isolated myself in order to prepare. At the time, I exhibited many cardinal signs of clinical depression. I never smiled. I suffered from what's called psychomotor retardation. My walking pace slowed. I wasn't sleeping well. For a time, my peripheral vision was even reduced. I felt like there was a cloud over my head. And while it was exciting to move to the big city, the tall buildings had an anxiety-inducing effect on me.

My oldest brother Phil was my lifeline during the first three tough months of my transition. I spoke to him a few times a week. During that time, he said to me something I've never forgotten: "You have to focus every minute of every day on your recovery." He told me to sleep more because it would give me the energy I needed to fight the stress. I did what my brother told me to do. He also told me I had to make a concerted effort to make friends in my new home. I committed to meeting someone new every day. I focused on developing new support systems. I joined a running group, and credit them with helping to bring me back to life. I met some truly amazing people in that group. They quite literally got me back on my feet.

The third time I went down was when I tried to live out my dream of owning a restaurant. Unfortunately, it was during the subprime mortgage crisis—the worst time in eighty years to open a new business. Additionally, I had no idea how to build or manage a restaurant, let alone deal with employees. Ultimately, the restaurant failed, and I stumbled again. I was ashamed. I felt like a failure. I didn't see my friends and family for an entire year. Finally, in the depths of another depression, I reached out to my brother Todd. He was a godsend. He helped me communicate with the vendors and my credit card company and negotiate solutions to my financial problems. My goal was to avoid filing for bankruptcy. I ended up selling the restaurant.

Stress is part of the human condition. It's the coping mechanisms and support systems that we develop that can get us through life's inevitable low points. Don't wait for a challenge to hit. Be proactive. Nurture relationships with good people every day. Support them and let them support you. Humans are social beings. We all get down from time to time and we need each other to help us get back up. Unfortunately, it took me three bouts with near depression to internalize that crucial life lesson, but I will never forget it.

If you are alone, reach out for support. There are good people everywhere—both inside and outside the health care system—and they will help you. You are never alone.

Excuses as a Roadblock

"It's cheaper to eat fast food than to cook a meal at home."

"I can't exercise because of my bad hip."

"I just can't find the time for a regular fitness routine."

There is a plethora of excuses we use to avoid putting our health front and center. Even the most disciplined among us occasionally have to combat excuses. It's human nature. But when you dig into many of the excuses we tell ourselves, they're total bunkum. Excuses are one of the biggest roadblocks on the journey to self-health and optimal well-being. It's easy to fall prey to them and accept them at face value. Honesty and frank self-assessment are requirements for achieving a state of wellness.

Take the fast food excuse. One of the worst things for your health is a poor diet. When your eating habits are unhealthy, you're more likely to get sick... and being sick is expensive. An illness might cause you to be docked pay at work or compel you to buy expensive medicines or pay for a doctor's visit. The money you think you're saving by having corn chips and a soda for lunch can quickly be eaten up by unforeseen medical bills (pun intended).

With regard to the bad hip, okay, maybe you can't run a marathon...but could you swim a few laps instead? The point is that you commit to some form of exercise. It's important for your health. Consider some of the daunting physical disabilities that the world's Paralympians face.

I hear it all the time from my patients: "Dr. G., I just can't find the time." Patients fighting diabetes or heart disease say it takes too much time to shop for healthier food, to exercise or schedule their annual wellness exams. My response is to explain what's at stake if they don't make their health a priority. The truth about the future they face is grim...and I don't hold back. After staring down this unhappy future, they are typically more open to the strategies for change that I have to offer. There are proven ways to deal with a busy schedule and put the "not enough time" excuse to rest.

Dr. G's Takeaways

- Fear, stress and loneliness are roadblocks. Don't let them prevent you from reaching your self-health goals
- Don't go it alone. Reach out to others to get you through life's tough times.
- Face your excuses. You have to in order to achieve health and wellbeing. We'll explore how in the next chapter.

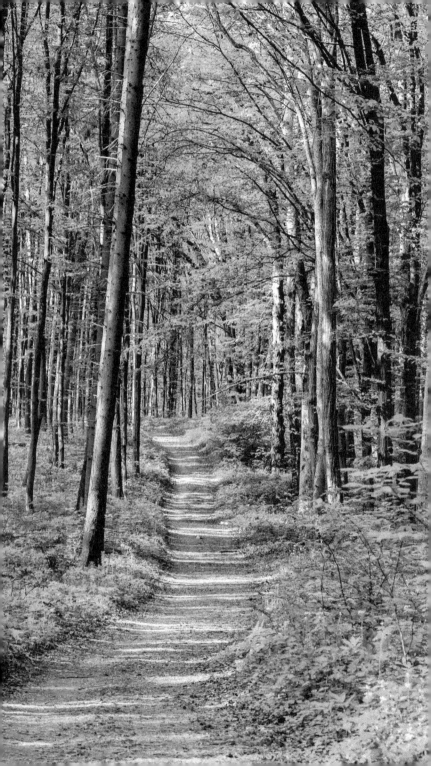

CHAPTER 3

Conquering Self-health Roadblocks

> *"The people who get on in this world are the people who get up and look for the circumstances they want, and if they can't find them, make them."*
>
> George Bernard Shaw, *Mrs. Warren's Profession*

A few years back, Duke University conducted a clinical research study that asked several thousand patients who were undergoing a cardiac diagnostic procedure what they thought about their likely future health. They followed these patients for fifteen years to see what happened to them. They found that the most optimistic patients were only about half as likely to die from heart disease as the most pessimistic ones. Mindset matters when it comes to health.

Mindset can be your ally or your enemy when you're trying to bring about change in your life. We all have days when we don't feel like sticking to the plan, even when we know it's good for our health. I sometimes struggle to muster up the energy to go to the gym before work or eat a vegetarian meal twice a week. Good days and bad days, ups and downs—these are a natural part of life. We get discouraged and want to give up. But the remedy for fear, stress, loneliness and excuses is hardiness, hope, support and hard work.

There are proven strategies to tackle life's challenges and overcome roadblocks to self-health. Here are a few that I recommend to my patients:

Start small

When you're getting started with a new health routine, set realistic, achievable goals. Instead of going to the gym five days a week, start with two days a week or even one day a week—maybe every Sunday afternoon. Pretty soon, you'll start seeing improvement in your health. Maybe a chunk of time will open up in your Wednesday evening schedule and can add a second workout session. As you gain confidence and find yourself in a positive rhythm, you can increase to three times a week, and later maybe even more. Start small and build.

Track your progress

We tend to improve the things that we measure, so track your progress. Get a calendar and put a big checkmark on it each time you execute a self-health task or goal—like keeping your calories low at dinnertime or going to the gym. As those checkmarks start to mount, they will motivate you. You'll be able to see at a glance how much time and effort you've invested in your self-health routines, and you'll be reluctant to let the momentum you've established evaporate.

Enlist a health buddy

The people around us have a great impact on our behaviors. Health buddies are people we enlist to help us stick to our self-health goals. When you decide to make a brisk evening walk part of your daily routine, consider scheduling it with a motivated friend or neighbor. It's much more motivating if you have someone else to go with you. You don't want to disappoint them by not showing up, so you show up. Also, it's good to share your goals with your health buddy. For instance, you might tell a health buddy, "I'm going to cut my drinking down and will only have alcohol on the weekend" or "I'm going to cut out sweets from my diet this month." If you make such a declaration to another person, you're much more likely to stick to your goal. We'll talk about health buddies in more detail later in the book.

Manage your time

Do you use the "not enough time" excuse? Then you need to find extra time in your busy day for health. There are some proven ways to do so. When you break it down, it's easier than you might think. You start by making a daily list and assigning priorities to the tasks on it. Then you identify ways to do those tasks more efficiently. Finally, you make a plan for managing life's interruptions.

Create a daily list

One of the best time-management tools that I use in my own life is the daily list. Some people dread their "to do" lists. Not me. Except when I'm on vacation, I create a list every single day. My list helps me keep my priorities straight and organize my day for maximum productivity and balance. I like to create my list the night before. The next morning, I briefly review it and am often surprised to see something I might have forgotten to do had it not been on my list.

When you're building your self-health plan, your list will be essential. It will motivate you and hold you accountable, and help you see patterns in your life that hold you back from achieving your goals. If, at the end of the day, the only thing not checked off your list is "sign up for the yoga class," it's going to pop. It's going to make you pause and think about why it didn't happen. Putting your health goals at the top of your list will change your life. Imagine how empowering it will feel when you can regularly check off items like "work out at 6PM," "eat 350-calorie lunch," "find vegetarian recipe for Saturday's dinner party."

Be realistic with your list. It may seem obvious— there are only so many hours in the day—but leave enough time to complete each of your tasks. Make sure you have everything to complete tomorrow's tasks ready in advance. This will set you up for success.

Prioritize your goals

A long list of goals can be overwhelming. You won't know where to begin. That's why prioritizing the items on your list is critical. I like to prioritize my health goals as either a 1, 2 or 3. A number 1 means the task absolutely must be done today. A number 2 tells me that it would be nice if I got to this task today, but it can wait until tomorrow. A number 3 is a task that I want to remember to do at some point in the near future.

A number 1 might be, "climb the five flights of stairs to my office." A number 2 could be "buy some zinc lozenges on my way home," and a number 3 would be something like "schedule a massage." This system of prioritization will make the list easier to manage. You know which items to start with, and if there are tasks that keep falling into the number 3 category, they can sometimes be combined, creating even more efficiency. For instance, all the health-related items you need to buy—like zinc lozenges, Band-Aids, vitamins, sunscreen—could be combined and picked up in one trip.

Now that you have a basic framework for how to prioritize your health and wellness tasks, it's important to look at the big picture in terms of what your priorities are for the week, month, or year. Our priorities are constantly shifting, so check in with yourself often. You can organize your list into different pages—one for today, one for this month, and one for this year.

It's helpful to rotate your priorities to give each one special attention. For example, if you've decided that you want to learn how to cook healthier meals, dedicate a week to making this a priority. You can break down this goal into smaller tasks and then prioritize those tasks on your daily list. For example, in order to learn how to cook healthier, you might dedicate a week to researching cooking classes and reading a book or two on nutrition. You'll also need to assess your schedule to figure out when you can fit grocery shopping and cooking into your schedule on a regular basis. If you want to live a healthier life, you'll need to put a variety of health and wellness tasks into your rotation of daily and weekly priorities—nutrition and weight management, exercise, stress management and relaxation.

Budget your time

It does no good to put tasks on your list if you don't have time to accomplish them. There's no point in adding a lofty wellness goal to your list if you know realistically that it won't happen. Not accomplishing the task or achieving a goal will only make you feel bad. The way to avoid this problem is to schedule the time and steps necessary to complete the task or achieve the goal. For example, if you put "stretching routine" on your list, add a time you intend to start the routine and the amount of time you will devote to it. Your entry might look like this: "stretching routine, 3-3:30 PM." Set a reminder on your calendar for this task. That way, when you're lost in your work day or daily routines, the reminder will help you remember. Over time, you won't need the reminder. The new task will become a routine.

You can also carve out more time for health and wellness by making changes to your schedule. If you truly feel like you have no time to exercise or cook a healthy meal, then prioritize a half hour to assess your current daily and weekly schedule. Maybe you're spending too much time at the office. In that case, perhaps you decide to have lunch at your desk and leave a half hour earlier. You could then use that half hour for a walk before dinner. Additionally, assess how you spend your leisure time. Do you watch a lot of television? Do you spend many hours on social media? Consider whether you could replace some of those passive activities with healthier pursuits like exercise, meditation or taking time to cook a healthy meal.

In your quest for self-health you need to budget for longer periods of downtime. Taking vacations is an essential practice of self-health. Whether that means an overnight stay at a downtown hotel or two weeks in Bali, getting away from your daily routine is crucial for rejuvenation. If your budget doesn't allow for that kind of vacation, consider a staycation. I'll give you some tips on that later in the book.

Delegate and outsource when possible

You've probably heard the common adage, "If you want something done right, do it yourself." Unfortunately, there are just too many tasks in our modern lives to do everything ourselves. That's why delegation and outsourcing are absolutely crucial if you want to achieve your health and wellness goals. Freeing up time for new daily health and wellness tasks and routines might require you to hire someone to clean your house or walk your dog. It's important to look at the daily workload from both your personal and professional life. Make a list of everything you do on a regular basis and research how much of it you might be able to delegate or outsource.

First, determine what your core competencies are and what is most important for you to do yourself. Just because you are able to do something, doesn't mean you should do it. If it's not a strength, you might want delegate. For example, many of us could learn to build our own websites, but is it worth the time and energy?

Many of us have a fear of losing control, which can manifest as a fear of delegating. We come up with excuses like, "I can do a better job myself" or "By the time I explain it to someone, I could have finished it myself." Getting real about our fears of losing control will help us be more open to delegating tasks.

Another common excuse is that delegating costs money. It's important to realize that your time also costs money. Think about it: if you spend hours doing something—say, for example, renting a machine and cleaning your carpets when you could pay a professional $125 to do them for you—it might take up a whole day. That's a day you could have used to go on a long bicycle ride and then attend a yoga class followed by cooking a healthy meal. Instead, you're too tired to do those things, so you go out to eat instead of cooking dinner for the family. You've squandered the money you saved.

And don't forget about technology. Using your bank's automatic bill payment system can save you many hours of check writing and mailing off bills. Keeping a shopping list on your mobile phone can save an extra trip to the grocery store for the bag of lemons you forgot to buy yesterday. You can change your recorded voicemail message to ask callers to suggest a good time to call them back, so you spend less time playing phone tag.

Avoid interruptions and distractions

A big part of time management is juggling life's inevitable interruptions. Over time, these distractions can impact our health. For example, you're researching treatment options for a skin condition and the phone rings. You forget about what you're doing and never gather the information you need to understand the condition. You're about to go for a run when a friend calls you. You take the call and ultimately never go for a run that day. When you're engaged in an activity related to your self-health plan, you're going to have to stay laser focused and create tactics to manage any interruptions that could interfere with your completing that activity.

Trying to multitask when working on a self-health goal is another form of distraction. What people usually mean when they use the word multitasking is task switching. People might believe they can pull this off, but frequently switching between various cognitive tasks has been scientifically proven to lower efficiency. You can get a lot more accomplished by fully completing one task before moving on to the next, so don't try to switch between a variety of tasks. Instead, focus completely on finishing the self-health task you have scheduled in the time period that you've set aside for that task. If you can master this focus, you'll see the benefits for the rest of your life.

Dr. G's Takeaways

- Face your health-related fears as the first step in overcoming them.
- Learn to deal with what's stressing you out and standing in the way of being well.
- Adopt an attitude of hardiness so you can better deal with stress.
- Take stock of whether loneliness is impacting your health.
- Enlist the support of others to overcome fears, stresses and loneliness.
- Combat excuses with facts.
- Manage your time to find extra time for healthful habits.

- Be realistic with your task list and allow enough time to complete each task before moving onto to the next one.
- As you become more time efficient, remember to fit in time for fitness and relaxation.
- Get support from a health buddy.
- Find alternative exercise routines to overcome limitations.

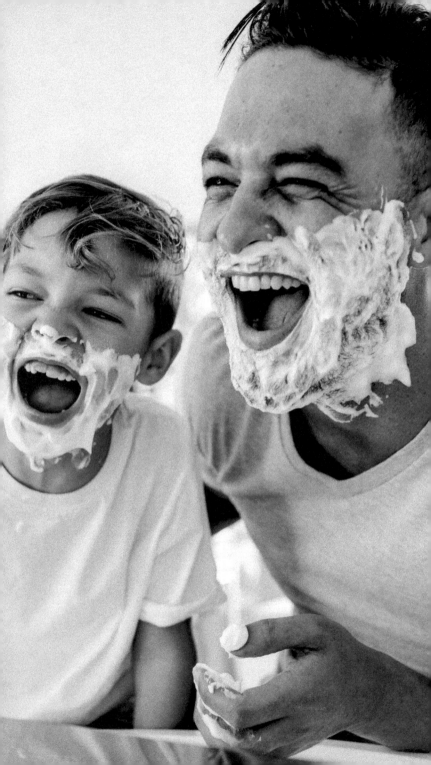

CHAPTER 4

Your Generation's Health-related Biases

> *"You have to have a cannon, so the next generation can come along and explode it."*
>
> Henry Louis Gates, American literary critic

We are all products of our times, and influenced by what others around us believe, say, and do. For example, studies have shown that if there is someone severely overweight in a cafeteria line, those in the line behind will eat more. Maybe they think, "I may be a little overweight, but I'm not as heavy as they are." Conversely, if our friends are constantly going to work out at the gym, we're more likely to do so ourselves. If we join them, it's even better. It's really important to see where we're getting our messages about wellness and what biases—whether our own or those of others—influence our behaviors.

So how do we start to identify biases and attitudes that keep us from prioritizing our health? My medical practice has patients of all ages—anywhere from age 18 to 104. Over the years, I've noticed that each generation has its own way of viewing and participating in the health care system. It occurred to me that a good place to start for anyone interested in uncovering their biases about health is to take a good look at the attitudes held by their generation. Doing so will provide insight into what may be worthwhile, and what might be standing in the way of good health. Let's take a look at how different generations approach health. This chapter will help you understand yourself better and help you find support in areas where you are weak.

1910 to 1924 - The Greatest Generation

Members of this generation experienced World War I. The automobile was just starting to change the way people lived. They were young adults during World War II and bore the brunt of fighting it. They came to believe in teamwork, patriotism, and the rewards of hard work. When it comes to their attitudes about health, they are firm believers in the authority of doctors and the medical system at large. Their health needs now are complex and often difficult. Although some people are living to be over one hundred, most of this generation has passed on. There are not many living members of this generation. Those who are still alive are mostly dealing with complex health and end-of-life issues.

1925 to 1945 - Traditionalists or Silent Generation

The traditionalists are also known as the silent generation. Like the previous generation, the silent generation lived through tough times, including the Great Depression and, for most of them, World War II. Like the generation before them, they became used to sacrifice and following orders. They are referred to as the silent generation because typically, they're quiet and don't make waves. The children of this era were expected to be seen and not heard. Today, they keep their feelings to themselves. Members of this generation have a strong work ethic and appreciate the value of working hard to reach their goals. They are the most trusting of the generations. They also honor their promises and commitments. Recognition is something this group values.

Traditionalists are often tough and have a stoic approach to their health. They respect authority, so they are more likely to trust the doctor and medical establishments when getting health information. This generation doesn't believe in overnight success, and this attitude can be beneficial because some health goals take a long time to achieve. They also tend to ignore important symptoms and postpone visits to their physician or push off trips to urgent care centers or emergency rooms, even as the symptoms become more severe. They are less likely to seek help if they have multiple conditions.

While trust is a positive characteristic, it can sometimes backfire. If a patient from the silent generation completely trusts his or her doctor to treat them, they might not ask to have their diagnosis explained. They are also less likely to ask important questions about a medicine or treatment's potential side-effects. I've seen this happen in my practice. Mary was in her late 60s when her husband Adam was hospitalized for tests. We discovered he had stage-four lung cancer, and probably not long to live. Needless to say, this was extremely difficult news for Mary to handle. "Dr. G.," she said. "Let's just not tell him. It will upset him. Just do what you think is best to treat him." Of course, I couldn't avoid telling Adam he had lung cancer. He had to be part of the decision-making process with regard to his treatment. How could Adam give informed consent if he didn't know his condition?

Traditionalists are the least likely people to initiate conflict at work or in relationships, and this can lead them to be reticent about discussing alternative medicines, procedures or surgeries.

They are apt to leave the doctor's office under-informed and potentially unprepared to deal with the health challenges they face.

One way that people from this generation can address these problems is to prepare a list of questions for the doctor before the visit. Another is to have a caregiver—a friend or family member from a different generation—accompany them to appointments. The caregiver can make sure the patient leaves with the information they need.

This silent generation is also less adept at using computers and modern technology. This is not surprising, since they were not brought up with tablets, cell phones, computers and smart televisions. As a result, they are less likely to have access to online resources and mobile apps that could help them with weight loss or fitness goals. Again, this is where a caregiver can step in, either by teaching them how to use digital tools or by doing important medical research online for them.

1946 to 1964 - Baby Boomers

The generation born after World War II grew up more privileged than previous generations. After decades of hardship, it was natural to celebrate. America became a more indulgence-oriented society. The "boomers" became accustomed to having more of everything. This attitude—combined with changes to the American diet, lifestyle and health care—has contributed to a new reality: 72 percent of men and 67 percent of women from this generation are now overweight or obese. The United Health Foundation reports that this generation will enter old age sicker than their parents did at the same age. They are plagued with diabetes and obesity, which can lead to heart conditions and other maladies. This is alarming news.

The baby boomers' weight problems are ironic, considering they also started a truly remarkable fitness revolution. Boomers brought us jogging, aerobics, and cardio fitness. In 1968, a best-selling book called *Aerobics* put this new form of exercise on the map. According to the AARP, from 1968 to 1984 the percentage of Americans who exercised regularly jumped from 24 to 59 percent. It's not surprising that deaths from heart disease dropped 48 percent over this same time period. Average life expectancy went from 69.7 years for those born in 1960 to 75.4 for those born in 1990. I find this to be strong evidence that cardio really does help prevent disease and leads to longer lives.

The same AARP study indicates the percentage of boomers working out regularly has fallen to 35 percent. Because of this generation's poor physical condition, they are more likely to get diabetes and have high blood pressure than their parents. What happened? Some believe economic, cultural and technological changes have changed the way boomers think about exercise. Some attribute it to our fast food diets.

The boomers are also a rebellious generation. They protested the Vietnam War and stood up for civil rights. They defied their conservative parents and created a more socially liberal lifestyle. The 1972 resignation of President Nixon after Watergate gave birth to this generation's strong distrust of government and other social institutions. They're less likely to trust their doctor's advice and more likely to seek alternative treatments like acupuncture or herbal medicines. With their strong belief that natural substances are the only thing that they should put in their bodies, they often see synthetic medicines as bad. While natural solutions play an important role in modern medicine, this generation's bias against prescribed medicines can sometimes have a negative impact on their medical treatment, especially for those who have been prescribed medicines to control diabetes or high blood pressure.

Boomers are notorious for their attempts to stay young. One of the generation's earliest sayings was, "Never trust anyone over 30." Now in their late 50s, 60s and 70s, they have had to reframe that idea. Many of them are still trying to stave off the effects of aging. They are the first generation to take part in anti-aging practices, buying skin care products, vitamins and supplements with some of them opting for Botox injections and even plastic surgery.

Most boomers I see in my practice tend to be optimistic and have a can-do attitude. Having experienced an improved quality of life and health, the thrill of starting a fitness revolution, is part of their collective memory. I always encourage them to call on the skills they developed earlier and return to a fitness regimen as the basis of their self-health program.

One of my patients, Bruce, embodies both the can-do attitude of the boomers and their commitment to fitness. I discovered that Bruce had high blood pressure, with the upper number 155. As I normally do, I suggested he reduce his blood pressure with relaxation techniques and a cardio program. Because he had a below-the-knee amputation of his right leg, he didn't think he could start a cardio program. I suggested swimming or using a rowing machine. Three weeks later when he came back to my office, I was spellbound by his results. His blood pressure had plummeted 30 points to 125. He told me that he had taken my advice and started using a rowing machine three hours a day, seven days a week. Any time I have a patient young or old who says they can't start a cardio routine due to some obstacle, I Bruce's inspirational story with them.

1965 to 1980 - Generation X

Sandwiched between two powerful and culture-changing generations, and covering a shorter time span, the Generation X population is small by comparison to their parents. Now in their forties and fifties, many individuals from this generation are becoming today's corporate leaders. Not only are they able to handle changes in technology, they are excellent problem-solvers, highly collaborative, and arguably the most entrepreneurial of any major group in the workforce today.

In the midst of juggling their careers, raising children, and often caring for aging parents, they have been called "the stress generation." To cope with life's pressures many have turned to playing videogames, consuming junk food, drinking, doing drugs and smoking. With the busy schedules and many daily pressures, the feel that something has to give. Often that means skipping their annual physical or follow-up visits for chronic conditions. Only about half of Gen Xers have had a physical in the last five years, compared to 70 percent of boomers. Only about four in ten do necessary health maintenance screenings.

Many Xers have moved into caregiver roles. This group consists primarily of women in their forties and fifties who take care of their parents, children and spouses. These caregivers often juggle responsibilities at work as well, making life balance a challenging pursuit. What usually suffers is their fitness routine and diet. This leads to problems of obesity, high blood pressure and the other pitfalls brought on by stress.

Generation Xers are also bearing the brunt of the increasingly high cost of health care. Given the fact that they are often the primary breadwinners in their extended families, they often have to help family members pay for medical treatments and medicines. Add nationwide disillusionment with the cost and access to health care, and you've got a perfect storm. En masse, this generation has opted out of preventative medical appointments and procedures. In a January 2018 report in *Forbes* magazine, it was noted that in the previous year almost half of Gen Xers didn't go to the doctor when they were sick or injured, 45 percent skipped a recommended medical test or treatment, and 40 percent went without a routine physical or other preventive health care. The reason? They didn't have the money.

1981 to 1996 - Generation Y or Millennials

The millennial generation is even larger than the boomer generation. Their formative years, included the tragedy of the 9/11 terrorist attack, the subprime mortgage crisis and economic downturn in 2009. Many millennials could not find jobs upon graduation from college; others found only low paying, unsatisfying employment. They also went to college at a time of rising costs, and many are saddled with huge amounts of college debt. To me, this generation seems more interested in work/life balance than Generation X. I think they seek this balance as a result of reexamining their values after facing so many crises and tragedies.

Millennials exercise more, smoke less and eat better than previous generations. They are very conscientious about their health and well-being. They are very open to technology assisted health trends like wearable health monitors and apps to monitor fitness and diet goals. With regard to acute and chronic pain, millennials are only half as likely as boomers to turn to opioids to manage their pain. Millennials—who search for motivation through social media and by sharing the latest medical, wellness and fitness technology trends—encourage each other to lead healthier lifestyles. Surveys show that 76 percent of this generation get exercise at least once a week. They're known for spending big money on gym memberships and health clubs.

One of the millennials' biggest accomplishments is bringing a greater food consciousness and awareness to society. Their eating habits have been a driving force behind the movement toward fresh, healthy and natural foods in the US. It's the millennials who have publicized—through social media and other means—the use of antibiotics in meats and the overuse of pesticides in our food. This is the generation that has compelled fast food chains to change where they source and prepare their food as well as what types of food they offer on their menu.

Six in ten millennials eat out at least once a week, and that's double what their boomer parents do. While studies have shown that eating out can have unhealthy consequences as to weight gain, at least millennials are more likely to patronize restaurants that serve less processed food, more cage-free eggs, antibiotic-free meats, organic and gluten-free products. Of all the generations, they're the most willing to pay a higher price for their food in order to receive the quality product they desire. This has a net positive impact on their health.

Millennials appear to have inherited the same deep distrust their boomer parents have for medical establishments, organizations, doctors, and hospitals. This strong bias often prevents them from logically discussing minor and major health issues when they come face-to-face with various health care professionals and/or health institutions.

Millennials have also been shown to have an unusually high diagnoses of anxiety and depression. I believe it may be because of their heavier use of social media, texting and Instagramming, which has cut down on the time they spend with others in person. Strong interpersonal relationships are a key factor in avoiding loneliness and depression.

Yet millennial's use of digital tools can have an upside. During a visit last year, I was very impressed by the research skills that Susan, one of my Millennial patients, displayed when she experienced mild diarrhea. Through online fact-finding, she discovered she should take probiotics and cultured yogurt to combat her symptoms. She did this, and her symptoms went away. At a more recent visit, she complained of a burning sensation during urination. Her symptoms indicated a urinary tract infection. However, she decided not to take antibiotics until her urine culture came back. In the meantime, she opted for cranberry pills. Only after her urine culture came back positive for the infection, did she agree to take an oral antibiotic. Susan had the discipline to do the right thing for her body. She educated herself, conferred with me, completed the necessary test, waited for the result and agreed to a necessary medical solution.

1997 to 2009 Generation Z

The oldest of this generation is just now coming of age. A discussion of this generation is included in this book primarily to help their parents and caregivers gain a better understanding of how to communicate with them about health.

They are the first generation to completely grow up in The Digital Age. They're known for their ability to multitask and quickly absorb snippets of information. They're resistant to receiving information that's not packaged in a way they like. Like the millennials, they are more likely to believe a hip, popular blogger with a large following than a spokesperson from health institution. Highly connected to a vast pool of online resources, they are less inclined to believe the information that doctors share with them. They are also skeptical about the health benefits of vaccines like the flu shot.

I thought I was being pretty hip and modern recently by showing one of my Gen Z patients the weight-loss app Lose It! that I have on my mobile phone. I pointed out how you can decide how many pounds to lose a week and track your progress. You can even scan the barcode of a food item and count the calories in the nutritional contents. My patient—an eighteen-old named Greg—took it all in. By the time I saw him again a few weeks later, he had the app all figured out. He showed me a fancy graph of his weight loss and how he had logged in an exotic international meal that he'd found on the Internet. In a few weeks, he was already using the app far more effectively than I had been using it after downloading it a year earlier.

How the Generations Can Help Each Other with Self-health

So now we have a sense of each generation's attitudes and practices regarding health. By seeking collaboration across generations, we can all benefit from a broader perspective on our health and well-being. Grandparents can show their millennial grandchildren how to cook satisfying recipes that they've spent a lifetime collecting. Millennials can advise their elders about how to substitute with healthier ingredients. Generation Xers can teach their older friends and family how to download and use wellness apps while boomers and Millennials can accompany elders to their doctor's appointments and research medications and alternative therapies for their grandparents' aches and pains...and so on.

By having a cross-generational conversation about health, members from each generation can learn to identify and manage their own biases—which are sometimes impediments to their self-health, wellness and medical care. It's worth taking a look at some of your own biases. What kind of attitudes are standing between you and a state of wellness? You have to see your biases in sharp detail before you can get serious about achieving self-health.

Dr. G's Takeaways

- The first step to optimal health is being honest with yourself.
- We must come to terms with personal biases that prevent us from achieving a healthy life.
- By understanding what influences our understanding of health and health care providers and institutions—family history, economic resources, upbringing and generation, among other things—we can reach out to others for health support in a more meaningful way.

PART 2

BUILDING STRONG HEALTH CARE RELATIONSHIPS

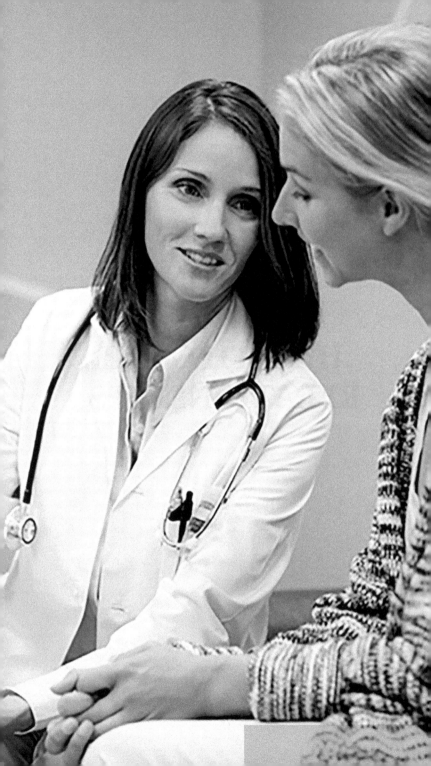

Finding the Right Doctor and Building a Simpatico Relationship

> *"The people who truly care about you won't have tell you they care; they'll show you."*
>
> Steve Maraboli, author, speaker, and behavioral scientist

When a patient calls me up at 10 o'clock at night and tells me about their abdominal pain, typically I can reassure them that it's not severe and suggest they follow up with me in a few days. On rare occasions, however, I have to tell them to go to urgent care or the hospital. In these cases, I call ahead and give the institution a heads up about my patient and their condition. If you are my patient, I have your back.

Most people desire a strong connection with their health care providers. They understand that an open, trusting doctor-patient relationship naturally leads to better health care outcomes. Why? Your health care provider knows you as a person. They understand your medical history. They understand when something is "off." That's not the case when you're dealing with a health care provider who doesn't know you. Conversely, when your doctor recommends a treatment, medication or lifestyle change, you know and trust them. You follow through on their recommendations because of that relationship. Nurturing this type of relationship with all the health care providers in your life is an essential component of any self-health plan. Why? Because self-health doesn't mean going it alone; it means championing your own health with the best knowledge, a positive mindset and a strong team of health care providers.

In today's world, however, this type of doctor-patient bond is more difficult to foster and maintain. Jobs frequently move health care providers around, and insurance can compel us to change doctors or practices. In spite of these and other challenges, it's important to nurture a close relationship with your health care provider whenever possible. In this chapter, I will show you how to find the right health care provider and foster a strong relationship.

Finding the Right Provider

Just like dating, it can take a while to find the right doctor. There will be a period of trial and error and a lot of "first dates" that lead nowhere. Before you begin your search, you'll want to understand clearly what you are looking for in a health care provider. There are more considerations then you might think. Here are some questions to ask yourself before you begin your research:

- Which health care provider groups does your insurance cover?
- If you opt for health care providers not covered by your insurance, do you have a budget to pay for those services?
- What types of accreditations would you like your health care provider to have?
- Is the location of the health care provider a priority?
- Do you require (or prefer) treatment by a doctor or are you open to meeting with a nurse practitioner or physician's assistant for some appointments?
- Is it important for health care provider to be available on a certain schedule?
- Is it crucial for your health care provider to have an affiliation with a hospital?
- What style of health care services are you looking for? Do want only in-person appoint-

ments or does the health care provider also need to offer telemedicine?

- What type of personality traits are you looking for your health care provider?
- What type of communications methods do you want them to offer—phone calls, texts, emails, or something else?
- What type of philosophy are you looking for in your provider? Do you prefer a western, holistic or integrative practice?

It's also important to understand that medical doctors can practice different types of medicine. There are a variety of credentials and philosophies when it comes to the style of care a health care provider offers. There are MDs who practice allopathic medicine, DOs who practice osteopathic medicine, and NDs who practice naturopathic or homeopathic medicine.

- **Allopathic medicine (MD)** is a healing system based on the logic that the way to fight off disease is by using an opposing force that confronts the illness head on. It relies on the scientific methods to extract from nature chemicals whose properties are intended to counteract the symptoms and overt physical manifestations of a given disease. The disease is considered to be no more than its physical manifestations. In most countries, MDs combine college and about six years of medical school. MDs train in hospitals and outpatient settings. Their extensive training in hospital settings can be an advantage in emergency situations. Another advantage to working with an MD is that they have often good relationships with a variety of medical specialists, such as dermatology, gynecology, and general surgery.

- **Osteopathic medicine (DO)** is a healing system in which the body is healed without any medicinal intervention. Only the hands of the physician (or needles) can balance the body's energies and realign it to its proper state. Osteopathic medicine includes Western chiropractic and Chinese acupuncture and acupressure. Like MDs, DOs go through training programs after medical school. They may enter an internship or residency program, which may be followed by subspecialty fellowship training. Their focus is on the entire patient: mind, body and spirit. They tend to be less about prescribing medicine and more about finding ways for the body to heal itself. DO's are fully licensed practitioners who can practice in all areas of medicine. They receive a unique training in musculoskeletal system.

- **Naturopathic medicine (ND)** is a healing system through which herbs and other resources are taken directly from nature. This system presupposes that there a natural cure for every disease—something that does not require human manipulation to alter its state. This healing system reflects a deep appreciation of the great, latent potential inherent in the earth. NDs receive training in a four-year program that includes basic medical sciences, nutrition, dietary supplements, botanical or plant medicine and other holistic remedies. They also employ acupuncture and lifestyle counseling. An advantage of going to a naturopathic doctor is his or her knowledge of natural healing agents. They use protocols that facilitate the body's inherent ability to restore optimal health. They tend to avoid prescription drugs whenever possible, though they do have knowledge about and sometimes utilize prescription drugs. Some of the most common conditions NDs treat are allergies, digestive issues, chronic pain and fatigue.

- **Homeopathic medicine (HD)** is recognized by the World Health Organization as the second most-practiced therapeutic system in the world. Though most popular in India and South America, there are millions of people throughout the rest of the world who adhere to the practice. Homeopathic treatment uses your body's own healing powers and relies on the minimal dose of any medicine given. Homeopathic medicines are gentle, subtle and powerful, and they are also non-addictive.

- **Chiropractic doctors (DC)** focus on the diagnosis and treatment of neuromuscular disorders with an emphasis on the treatment through manual adjustment and or possibly manipulation of the spine. Their goal is typically to decrease pain and improve function and range of movement. They recommend exercises and other therapies to decrease pain. They are also skilled in ergonomics—the use of devices to strategically improve joint function.

After you fully understand the type of health care provider you want and the qualities of that provider that are important to you, then it's time to begin your search. For most people, the easiest place to start is the available network of providers offered by your insurance. Most insurance companies allow you to search for in-network providers based on location. Unless you're searching for a very niche specialist or nontraditional provider, beginning your search in network is usually a natural first step.

No matter whether you choose and MD, DO or NP, each will have their own individual philosophy. When you have your first meeting, you'll want to ask each health care provider their philosophy of medicine—whether holistic, western or integrative. You'll also want to understand each doctor's reputation with patients. How can you dig deeper while ensuring you get unbiased, third-party reviews and testimonies? There are a number of reputable search tools available.

- **consumerreports.org.** Many health care providers are affiliated with hospitals. Their relationship can dictate which hospital you'll go to in emergency situations. You can search provider hospital affiliations at consumerreports.org/health/hospitals/ratings

- **certificationmatters.org.** If a health care provider is certified by the American Board of Medical Specialties (ABMS), you know they have a degree from a reputable medical school, have completed the required residency training, passed a number of ABMS exams, and are licensed by the state. They're also held to continuing medical education requirements. You can search for board certified providers at certificationmatters.org

- **webmd.com.** Though WebMD has its limitations with regard to helping people accurately diagnose illness based on their symptoms, it offers an incredibly thorough and reliable list of health care provider ratings and testimonies. WebMD can provide a fairly comprehensive look at a doctor's reputation. Visit doctor.webmd.com

- **healthgrades.com.** One of the most well-known third-party tools to search for doctors and view testimonies and ratings, this site helps millions of people each month find and make appointments with healers. By partnering with over 500 hospitals around the country there might be some bias, but they also have a wide circle. Get a more holistic view of potential healers by visiting healthgrades.com.

If you're looking for a non-traditional provider—such as an acupuncturist, homeopathic, or naturopathic doctor—your insurance company may not cover services provided by these types of specialists or offer information about them (since they are most likely out of networks). That's where searching by hospital affiliation, relevant board certifications based on their specialty, and sites like WebMD and Healthgrades can help.

Whether you're searching for traditional or non-traditional providers, it's good to start by scheduling a consultation—that "first date" we talked about earlier. Actually, it's more like a job interview—and you're the one doing the hiring. Just because a provider looks good online doesn't mean they're the best fit for you. Your instincts during the interview are just as important (if not more so) than the health care provider's online presentation and credentials.

As you start your consultation with a number of health care providers, be honest with yourself not only about what you *want* in a doctor, but what you *need* as well. As I've mentioned, it's important to find health care providers who will actively listen, challenge ideas when necessary, and advise in a forthright manner. Your health care provider should be someone with whom you can build a strong professional relationship for many years to come. Early detection and prevention are the best approaches to health and wellness. Not only does this require a good diagnostician, it takes a strong communicator who is willing to be frank with you about symptoms and unhealthy lifestyle choices as well.

You may not find a health care provider that you connect with on your first, second, or even fifth meet-and-greet. Don't get discouraged, you're learning. With each interaction, you'll discover a bit more about what you're looking for in a health care provider. Jot down a few notes after each consultation. What worked? What was missing? This will help guide you towards the right relationship.

Fostering Strong Relationships with Your Health Care Provider

Once you find the right health care provider, it's time to start strengthening your connection. A solid doctor-patient relationship must be built on mutual respect, honesty, transparency, compassion, and empathy. Building this rapport takes time and effort from both parties. For a lot of people, however, seeing a doctor dredges up feelings of worry. They are on edge the minute they walk into a doctor's office. When you're not looking forward to an encounter, it's difficult to build rapport. Health care providers can usually sense these things, compounding the problem. Think about it—would you be excited to see someone if you knew they were dreading the encounter with you? Probably not.

Overcoming these emotional obstacles will take a concerted effort. Remember, like you, your health care provider is only human. Mindfully practicing basic graces can work magic. Embrace kindness, compassion, empathy and gratitude during your first encounter. Set the tone and expect your health care provider to return this good energy. Know that there will be some days when one or both of you are just a little "off." Understand your communication preferences and dedicate yourself to building a relationship with a health care provider who has the same preferences.

Effective Use of Email, Phone, Text, or Telemedicine with Your Healer

Clear and effective communication between you and your health care provider is paramount for a good relationship. You won't be able to achieve your health and wellness goals without it. In this digital era, there are numerous new ways to communicate with your doctor. To compliment your in-person appointments, you can now commonly email, call or text your providers. May practices also now offer telemedicine, which allows you to visit or check in with your doctor virtually through screen-sharing technologies such as Skype.

Each communication method has its pros and cons. How many times have you had a misunderstanding with a friend, partner, or family member because your tone couldn't be properly conveyed by a text message? A similar issue can occur with your health care provider when texts or emails are the method of communication you're using. Even telemedicine has its limitations. Often it isn't possible for a doctor to diagnose a condition remotely—even if he can see you on camera. In these cases, you'll still need an in-person appointment for proper treatment.

Still, telemedicine *can* be very helpful and convenient in many situations. Sometimes, it may be the *only* way to communicate with your health care provider. For instance, if you are immobilized and/or live in a rural or remote area where it is difficult to find health care providers. For others, telemedicine can help "fill in the blanks" between in-person appointments.

Dr. G's Takeaways

- Before you start searching for a health care provider, understand what qualities and services you want from your provider.
- Start your search in-network, if possible, and check out various impartial ratings and information sites.
- Don't be afraid to schedule several "dates" or consultations with potential providers.
- Work to build a strong, long-term relationship with your health care provider. This will require mutual respect, honesty, transparency, compassion, and empathy.

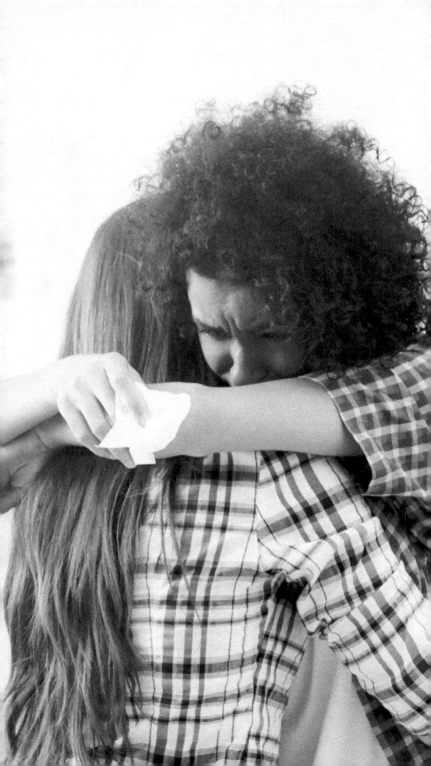

CHAPTER 6

Finding and Nurturing Support

> *"Nurturing has the ability to transform people's lives."*
> *John C. Maxwell, bestselling American author*

"No man is island..." begins the famous poem by John Donne. People all over the world quote this famous poem because there is immense truth in this message. As I mentioned earlier in the book, there were three critical times in my life where I needed a lifeline. I reached out to family and friends in my times of need. During those times, it was an immense comfort to know others were there to support me. I was not alone. These amazing people pulled me through some very rough times. These experiences shaped me both personally and professionally. I know firsthand the importance of nurturing a health care support community and turning to them in times of trouble. You need to build and nurture a team of supportive people—both inside and outside the health care system—to assist you in your self-health journey. Some of the people on this team will be there to provide emotional support; others can assist with physical illnesses; and still others can provide information or administrative support—like taking notes when you visit a specialist, finding a reliable online resource to learn more about a medical condition or navigating an insurance claim.

Health buddies

I define the term "Health Buddy" as anyone who supports you in achieving your health goals. When setting your health and wellness goals—refer to Chapter One if you need a refresher—define your weakest area and find a health buddy to motivate you and hold you accountable.

I want my patients to achieve their health goals, so a few years ago I began pairing them up with health buddies within their families. I've continued this practice because it works. If one family member is talented in physical fitness, I pair them up with a family member who is fitness challenged or lacks the motivation to work out. If another family member is trying to lose weight, I pair them up with someone in their family who has successfully lost and kept off weight or who has a strong understanding of nutrition. A smoker in the family might get a health buddy who has already quit or one who lives a healthy lifestyle, free of such addictions.

A health buddy serves as a witness to your health goals and can help you reach milestones on your way to success. They can motivate you and remind you how good you feel when you achieve your health goals. They are your self-health partner. When things go off track—as they inevitably will sometimes—your health buddy is there guide you back toward your health and wellbeing goals.

A health buddy needs to be someone who can be honest with you, who can speak frankly when you're not achieving your goals. Whether they are a family member, friend or colleague, there needs to be a high level of trust and respect between you and your health buddy. During the three toughest times in my own life, I relied on a health buddy for help. One time, I relied on a fellow medical student for support; two other times, I turned to my brothers, who were a lifeline during two challenging transitions in my life. I listened to what they had to say, even when they were telling me to do things that seemed challenging. I wouldn't have made it through without their advice, and occasional "tough love." If you are serious about creating and sticking to your self-health plan, you'll want to find at least one—if not several—health buddies.

Caregivers

I was surprised when I learned that four out of ten adults in the U.S. are caregivers—that is, someone who provides assistance to someone else who is ill or to some degree incapacitated. There are about fifty million informal and family caregivers providing assistance to the chronically or acutely ill and disabled persons. About nine million caregivers care for someone fifty or older who has dementia.

While it is estimated that about sixty-five to seventy percent of caregivers are women, an increasing number of men are now playing the role of caregiver. The average age of the family caregiver is forty-five. The average age of those caring for someone sixty-five or older is sixty- three, and about a third of those caring for that age demographic are in poor health themselves. About forty percent of the time, the patient's child is the caregiver. Twenty five percent of the time, it's another relative who plays this role, and roughly twenty percent of the time a spouse is doing the caregiving. About half of all caregivers have a full-time job, and another ten percent work part-time. When they come home, they face another full-time job taking care of their loved ones. They deserve our respect and gratitude.

In my years of medical practice, I have come across some stellar caregivers. They are an important part of a patient's health care team—masters at handling the many daily tasks that the patient can no longer manage on his or her own. They cook meals, bathe patients, make sure the patient's bills are paid, purchase supplies, schedule doctors' appointments, and administer necessary medicines. Over time— through their diligence in learning from primary care professionals and specialists, physical therapists, wound care, nurses and others—caregivers often develop an innate understanding of their patients' needs and acquire specialized knowledge about how to take care of their problems.

The Pew Research Center studied family caregivers and their use of technology. They found that the caregivers were very much engaged in the pursuit of health information and support care advice, both online and in person. The information they gathered online was particularly helpful for researching the patient's medical problems, treatments, and drugs. They also gather health information from non-medical people, including family, friends, and clinicians. When caregivers visit my office, I'm often impressed by their ability to cite a litany of valuable information and accomplishments. They know every ticket each specialist gave them, can list the dates of every upcoming appointment, share details on all medications, talk about how they got a bill covered by insurance after weeks of persistence, and describe all their patient's daily health routines.

As you might be able to tell, I have tremendous respect for caregivers, and I'd like to share a few stories to demonstrate the crucial role they can play in a patient's health care support network:

Lina — Coordinating Care

Juan had been in a crippling accident that left him with fractures, leg contracture, and vision and hearing difficulties when he was run over by a garbage truck and dragged for two blocks in the underpinning. Many of his injuries have never healed properly. His girlfriend Lina diligently stepped in to stay on top of Juan's injuries, surgeries, medicines, and many specialist appointments, from orthopedists to eye doctors.

I have known Lina for the last five years and have been truly impressed by her commitment in making sure than Juan gets to all the important appointments necessary for his care. Every time she visits, she gives me detailed reports about Juan's other visits with the specialists.

When the Affordable Care Act was first introduced four years ago, Juan's coverage contracted.

Lina was frustrated that Juan could no longer go to certain specialists that he needed. She researched the insurance market to find an insurance product that would cover all the doctors currently caring for Juan. She ultimately found a plan that would allow Juan to continue to see all of his key doctors as well as his primary care doctor—me.

Juan went through a period of depression and gained twenty pounds. I told them both that it was important for Juan to lose this weight. Lina became an incredible taskmaster over his diet choices until he lost the weight. To my astonishment, just six weeks later, he had lost the entire twenty pounds.

Another time, Juan became suicidal. Lina got him to the needed emergency crisis services, and now makes sure he gets to his psychiatrist regularly. Lina knows every single medication Juan needs to take, including their dosage and frequency. She knows which medicines need to be refilled as well as their potential side effects. Sometimes talking with Lina is like talking to one of my medical colleagues.

Lina keeps a medical appointment book and list of medicines. She presents these to me at every appointment. She faithfully tells me about each specialist's recommendations and makes sure I record them in Juan's chart. As a primary care doctor this is extremely helpful. I don't have to call the specialist's office to track down this information. Lina has developed a strong rapport not only with me, but also with Juan's specialists. She is able to capture the key takeaways from each visit, understand them, and apply them to help Juan. She wants to make sure all-important information is relayed to me, both for continuity's sake and to get my opinion on Juan's progress.

Juan has a complex set of long-standing orthopedic injuries or bone fractures, and a condition where the muscles and tendons in his legs are shortening, which leads to rigidity of his legs. As a long-term care doctor, I often see the cycle of going back-and-forth from the nursing home to the hospital due to bedsores and/or other complications. Lina's strength as the caregiver has helped prevent Juan from needing multiple possible admissions and a nursing home stay.

Sara — Providing Emotional Support

I first met Robert when I was on call one night at St. Mary's hospital in Chicago. After a difficult tour of duty in Iraq, he began using heroin to cope with the stress. Thin and anxious, he was admitted with a severe bone infection called osteomyelitis, which was caused by his drug abuse. He needed surgery to remove part of his infected collarbone. He came through the surgery without incident and was dispositioned to go to a long-term care hospital to complete six weeks of antibiotics.

Robert was alone until his sister Sara stepped in. She wanted to help her brother face his heroin addiction and recover fully from his surgery. She often left Robert gifts to encourage him and let him know that he was loved.

Sara was there when I told Robert the hard truth. "You're malnourished, depressed and have a bone infection. Heroin is going kill you. You must stop using heroin now." In a very military fashion, Robert replied, "You have my word, as a man. I will not ever do heroin again."

I learned a couple months later how Sara had helped Robert become drug-free. She had taken care of his wounds and was always there for him to talk with and to help him find the support he needed. As a result, Robert is now adapting well to civilian life. Although he had two drug relapses after his hospital stay, he eventually quit using heroin and has been clean for more than two years. Sara's willingness to get involved helped Robert start the healing process. She helped him remember the person he was before the war and guided him back to being that person again.

Anna — Stroke Care

Anna's brother Benjamin suffered a stroke at age sixty-six. It left him weak on the left side, unable to talk, and subject to frequent seizures. When we see older people suffer a stroke, we're often faced with a poor prognosis and sometimes a downward spiral in the health condition leading to bad outcomes like falls, fractures, bedsores, pneumonia and infection. That's why caregiving after a stroke is so challenging. Anna rose to the challenge. Most all of Benjamin's deficits were eventually restored. He was speaking and walking, and was put on seizure medications, which were only adjusted once. He has not had a seizure, and while he has maintained a mild residual weakness from the stroke, he has been walking well for the last five years.

An important side-note for those who have been struggling with a stroke victim: one of my patients was a former U.S. Senator from Illinois, Mark Kirk. Mark had a stroke that he famously recovered from eventually walking up the U.S. Capitol steps with the support of his good friend, Senator Joe Manchin of West Virginia. I was told it was unlikely Mark would ever walk again. He was quoted in the *Chicago Tribune* saying just two words: "Rehab works." I often try to motivate my patients in the rehab process using this story because many of them know of Mark Kirk. Yes, physical rehab does work. I've seen this kind of recovery hundreds of times for those who motivate themselves or have the good fortune of a caregiver like Anna.

Rosa and Luis — Reciprocal Caregivers

Rosa was young and energetic. She worked out and didn't expect that her high blood pressure or high cholesterol were a serious issue. Then, she suffered a heart attack at age thirty. Her boyfriend was at her side when it happened. Luis helped Rosa get back on her feet with a proper diet, exercise and blood pressure and lipid-lowering medications.

A couple of years later, Luis lifted a cordon of steel at his job and painfully twisted his back. The torsion injury caused a herniated disc and spinal stenosis. He ended up with severe pain and in need for neurosurgery. Rosa helped Luis fill out all the proper forms needed to battle his Workmen's Compensation claim. It took over a year, but finally Workmen's Comp agreed to cover all his medical costs. Luis lost his job and there were tough times for the couple. Rosa remained by Luis' side the whole time. She helped to facilitate the required consensus from the medical community, including myself as his primary care doctor. A neurologist, a neurosurgeon, and I all agreed that he had a work-related injury and qualified for Workmen's Compensation.

After the surgery Rosa helped Luis get to the sports medicine doctor for evaluation and set up sports-specific physical therapy. I continued to see them both as a couple. Rosa would help Luis relate the stories of his battle with pain and loss of function. They were both doing well. Rosa and Luis show us the benefits of reciprocal caregiving.

Supporting your support system

Being a caregiver can be very stressful, especially in situations where a loved one suffers from a serious medical condition like dementia. I have seen the stress in my patients who are caregivers. Sometimes they are hesitant to talk about this stress, but I encourage them to seek counseling when the burden gets to be too great.

There is ongoing research to help address the issue of caregiver stress and burnout. Due to the growing number of people in the U.S. playing the role of caregiver, the subject has been written about extensively. The good news is that a lot of caregivers are able to recognize the signs of burnout and seek help. Because caregivers know the medical system better than most, they're able to navigate the system to get help when needed. Unfortunately, due to their focus on others, caregivers are also often the last to seek help for themselves. The Family Caregiver Alliance's National Center on Caregiving, (caregiving.org) is a very supportive and knowledgeable organization that has amazing online resources for caregivers.

If you have a caregiver helping you or a loved one, make sure to support them and show them your gratitude. The same with the health buddies in your life. These people have invested time and effort to support you. Nobody likes the friend who only calls when they're in trouble. Don't be that person. You shouldn't contact your self-health support team only when you're sick or stressed out. When you are doing well, reach out to them and return the favor or you're your gratitude. Get them a card or treat them to dinner. It doesn't have to be expensive, just something that acknowledges your appreciation of their support.

It's important to support your support system. Think of this like an emotional bank account. Whenever you can, make a deposit of kindness and gratitude. When they are in need, be sure to show them the same loving support they gave to you when you needed it. There are even health benefits associated with giving to others. An article in *Greater Good* magazine sums it up well:

> A wide range of research has linked different forms of generosity to better health, even among the sick and elderly. In his book *Why Good Things Happen to Good People*, Stephen Post, a professor of preventative medicine at Stony Brook University, reports that giving to others has

been shown to increase health benefits in people with chronic illness, including HIV and multiple sclerosis.

A 1999 study led by Doug Oman of the University of California, Berkeley, found that elderly people who volunteered for two or more organizations were 44 percent less likely to die over a five-year period than were non-volunteers, even after controlling for their age, exercise habits, general health, and negative health habits like smoking. Stephanie Brown of the University of Michigan saw similar results in a 2003 study on elderly couples. She and her colleagues found that those individuals who provided practical help to friends, relatives, or neighbors, or gave emotional support to their spouses, had a lower risk of dying over a five-year period than those who didn't.

We'll talk more about "paying it forward" in an upcoming chapter. Suffice to say, though, the old adage "it is in giving that we receive" is not to be taken lightly. Support your self-health support team, including any caregivers and health buddies in your life. They are special people who have been there for you in the tough times. They deserve your kindness and gratitude.

Dr. G's Takeaways

- Health buddies can motivate you, hold you accountable and help you achieve your self-health goals.
- The best caregivers develop an innate under-standing of their patients' needs and acquire specialized knowledge about how to take care of their problems.
- Remember to support your support system. Say "thank you" often and be there when they need you.

вейте Hola سلام د

ัสดี

ちは

lo

uton

allo Ahoj

a Salve

Përshëndetje

Dia duit

Привет

नमस्ते

Sveiki

вствуйте

Salam

pari Γεια σας

Bonjou హల్లో

CHAPTER 7

Demystifying the Health-Care System

> *"Without translation, we would be living in provinces bordering on silence."*
>
> George Steiner, American-French literary critic

Information is key when you're practicing self-health. Understanding how the health care system works and how to navigate it is important and can lead to better health outcomes. But between health care specialties, different types of providers and medical facilities...it can be a maze. There's a lot to learn. If you need to see multiple doctors for advice or treatment, you are likely to encounter different questions and processes at each provider. You might be subjected to testing in sprawling medical facilities that seem foreign. When you get a lab test, you might not be totally sure why or for what you're being tested. Your test results might not be explained to you fully...and if they are, you might not always understand what you're being told. It's a lot to navigate, especially when you're not feeling well or concerned about your symptoms. Relax! Dr. G is here to demystify the health care system, so you can better understand the facilities you visit, the personnel with whom you speak, and make sense of the test results and medical advice that you receive.

Types of Facilities

Let's begin by learning about the different type of medical facilities. We'll start with pharmacies and work our way up through doctors' offices, medical clinics, urgent care centers, emergency rooms and hospitals. We'll also have a look at telemedicine portals where you can participate in health care virtually.

Pharmacies

Pharmacies are locations for dispensing medication—both generic and brand name. You probably already know this. However, did you know that many pharmacies also now provide some immunizations and health screenings as well as carry vitamin and mineral supplements and some herbal and holistic remedies? In the U.S., most pharmacies are located in drugstores, which also sell common over-the-counter medications amid a host of other items. However, there are other locations for and types of pharmacies. Hospitals and walk-in clinics also often have pharmacies. There are independent pharmacies that aren't associated with drugstores or chains. They usually have fewer customers, and therefore, shorter wait times. Finally, there are compounding pharmacies, which prepare personalized medications for patients. Compounded medications are made based on prescriptions that require the pharmacist to mix individual ingredients in the exact strength and dosage required by the doctor to treat your illness. In all of these settings, the mission of the pharmacy has expanded in recent decades. In the next section, you'll learn about how some pharmacies are even being turned into medical clinics. It's worth looking into what your local pharmacies have to offer.

Though you can't negotiate the price of your medications at a pharmacy, there is often a generic version of the requested drug. Often, generic versions of a medication are significantly cheaper than the brand-name version. It's always worth asking your pharmacist about this option. However, if your pharmacist does not recommend a generic drug, ask them why. There might be a very good reason for their decision. Not all generic drugs are exactly the same as their brand name counterparts. Directions to not use a generic version of a medication might be indicated on the prescription from your doctor or suggested by the pharmacist. If this is the case, it's best to heed their advice.

Outpatient primary care centers

Outpatient primary care centers are facilities that serve day-to-day health care needs. You can go here to meet with your primary care physician, get a routine physical, and tend to non-emergency medical concerns. Outpatient primary care centers do not provide overnight medical care. They come in several shapes and sizes. Here is a short list of the most common types of outpatient primary care centers:

Doctors' offices

Generally speaking, a doctor's office is the private practice of one or more primary care physicians. To visit a doctor's office, you need to make an appointment. Sometimes the appointment schedules of the doctors in a practice are filled and you have to wait several hours or longer for an appointment. If time is a factor, a medical clinic might be a better option for minor or standard medical conditions. There is usually a shorter wait time at a clinic. On the flip side, most patients find that the quality of care at a doctor's office is top notch. You can also develop a stronger relationship with a doctor that you see many times, and as I've already mentioned, this has numerous advantages. They know you and your medical history.

Medical clinics

Clinics are known for being accessible, affordable, and convenient. There are different types of clinics—retail clinics, urgent care clinics, free clinics, and community health clinics. The quality of care varies at clinics, so it's important to do your research.

In 2000, Minute Clinic (a division of CVS pharmacy) launched the first walk-in clinic in the U.S. to be located inside a national-chain drugstore. The main appeal of this type of clinic is the ability to go to your local drugstore and see a nurse or physician on the spot without an appointment. While retail clinics rate high on convenience, they do have some limitations. Clinics are not an adequate replacement for a primary care physician or pediatrician. They are not recommended for small children. Doctors at a clinic do not have your medical history on hand, which puts them at a significant disadvantage in diagnosing your medical issue. Additionally, since you rarely see the same doctor twice at a medical clinic, they eliminate the possibility of maintaining a long-term relationship. Though many people use medical clinics for their primary care, in my opinion they can't replace the advantages of having a long-term relationship with a primary care physician for all the reasons stated in early sections of this book. However, if you're looking to get a flu shot or medicine to treat the common cold, a clinic can be an excellent option.

Urgent care centers

This type of clinic focuses on ambulatory or walk-in services. It's for patients who require immediate care for an injury or illness that is not serious enough to warrant a visit to the emergency room but can't wait for a doctor's office schedule to open up. Most urgent care centers have onsite diagnostic equipment and can perform minor medical procedures.

Unlike medical clinics, urgent-care centers are usually staffed by one or more physicians who is typically trained in family or emergency medicine. Urgent care clinics also typically offer more services than medical clinics. For example, they often have the equipment to diagnose and treat broken bones and deep cuts that require stitches. More involved procedures and surgeries need to be treated in a hospital.

Emergency department

Sometimes referred to as ERs, emergency rooms are usually located in hospitals. These treatment facilities specialize in acute care, which means the patient receives active but short-term care for a severe injury, serious episode of illness, or urgent medical condition. These facilities are not designed to care for chronic, or ongoing, conditions. If you are in a car accident or battling a severe case of the flu, you might visit your local ER.

Most emergency departments operate twenty-four hours a day, seven days a week. A major part of ER care is prioritization. Depending on how emergency room doctors prioritize your case, you may be seen immediately or end up sitting in a waiting room for a very long time while cases deemed more urgent are treated. To decrease the uncertainty of wait time, some emergency rooms have adopted text services, so patients can keep their place in line and be notified when they get to the front.

Hospitals

At a hospital, you'll find a medical and nursing staff as well as specialized equipment. There are general hospitals that typically have an emergency room and specialized hospitals such as children's hospitals, psychiatric hospitals, trauma centers, and geriatric hospitals. Many hospitals have a variety of departments such as radiology, cardiology, and surgery. Hospitals typically treat both outpatients and inpatients (those who stay overnight).

To make your experience as seamless as possible, most hospitals now have all the registration paperwork available to fill out online. You can download the forms and complete them before you arrive. When you visit a hospital, remember to bring at least one form of identification—your insurance card, social security card, license, etc.—as well as a notebook to write down important information. You might also consider bringing some form of payment, in case a service or procedure is not covered by your insurance.

Telemedicine Portals

Partly in response to growing medical costs and a population that demands more convenience, telemedicine portals continue to gain popularity. These portals provide online access to doctors, counselors, psychiatrists or dermatologists via mobile app, video and/or phone. You can schedule appointments, upload or download medical data and images, and even have online video consultations with doctors. The costs are much lower than a trip to the emergency room or even the family doctor. Telemedicine portals are an increasingly important health care tool for those who wish to practice self-health. An example of a telemedicine portal is mdlive.com, which lets you sign up and talk to a doctor at any time—twenty-four hours a day, seven days a week.

Types of Medical Personnel

The cast of characters in health care is large. Each player seems to do their own thing. Often, communication between providers can be limited.

I want to help you demystify what the different professionals do, what services they can and can't provide for you, and what these professionals need in order to assist you effectively.

Certified nursing assistants (CNAs)

One of the most hands-on personnel you will interact with in the health care system, CNAs are found in nursing or residential care facilities and occasionally in hospitals. CNAs are responsible for the intimate day-to-day tasks of caring for you. This care can include bathing, dressing, feeding, cleaning rooms, dressing wounds, emptying bedpans, taking vital signs, and repositioning/turning. A CNA is under the direct supervision of a registered nurse.

A CNA may have a lot of experience interacting with patients, which is why they are often the first to notice health changes. However, they are not typically as knowledgeable on specific medical conditions as a doctor or nurse. A CNA is not required to have a bachelor's degree. Some CNAs complete four to twelve-week certification programs and have passed state exams before starting their careers; others have not.

Nurses (RNs)

Sometimes referred to as a registered nurse or RN, nurses have many responsibilities. Depending on the setting, a nurse might be responsible for administering medication, assisting physicians with medical procedures, monitoring patients, educating patients and their family members, completing assessments, and facilitating admissions and discharges. Nurses may also handle follow-up tasks such as scheduling MRIs and Xrays or setting up appointments with specialists.

When multiple institutions or doctors are involved in your diagnosis and/or treatment, nurses often manage the communication—passing information between physicians, specialists, families, and CNAs. Many times, they are the liaison between you and the doctor when you're in the hospital. The nurse is usually the key person on your medical team who has the most complete view of your entire health situation. They will know your medications, what tests have been ordered, which family members are involved in your care, and the names of all your doctors and specialists.

Not all nurses work in hospitals. Approximately forty percent of nurses can be found in clinics, physician's offices, schools, assisted living facilities, and homes. Nurses can also specialize in such areas as heart care, family practice, pediatrics, geriatrics, midwifery, labor and delivery, and emergency nursing. It's in your best interest to communicate as much as possible with your nurse because he or she will then pass that information onto the rest of your medical team and your family. Your nurse will keep everyone in the loop.

Nurse Practitioners (NPs)

Nurse practitioners and physician's assistants (PA) work under doctors and also function relatively independently. They often specialize in one area of medicine like adult primary care geriatrics, pediatrics or gynecology. They diagnose and treat illnesses, educate about conditions, perform physicals, and order or perform diagnostic tests. They can also prescribe and administer certain medications. Specific functions will vary depending on the state in which they practice.

For routine medical care, an NP or PA can perform most necessary services. Even though these health care providers don't have an "MD" after their name, they have gone through extensive medical training, including earning a master's degree. If you have an obscure medical condition that is difficult to diagnose or you need a surgical procedure, you'll want to see a doctor. Otherwise, an NP or PA is often able to treat you.

Primary care doctors (MDs, DCs, DOs, NDs, HDs)

These health care providers are typically the first stop whenever you sense something is wrong with your health. They oversee routine checkups, diagnose illnesses, come up with treatment plans, prescribe medications, and direct patients to specialists when appropriate.

As part of your self-health program, it's very important to have a primary care physician, even if you're not sick. Building a long-term relationship with your primary care physician increases the likelihood that you will get a correct diagnosis and the best treatment when something goes wrong. A good primary care physician can play a key role in preventive care by educating and coaching you during your regular checkups. Developing a partnership for prevention will keep you well and restore balance when you are not well. To learn more about the different types of primary care physicians, refer to Chapter Five.

Specialist physicians

This group does exactly what their name suggests— they specialize in a particular area of medicine. In order to specialize, they've had very specific education and clinical training in one area of health care. There are countless types of specialists, but a few examples are obstetricians, dermatologists, cardiologists, gynecologists, Immunologists, pediatricians, and psychologists.

Most insurance plans require you to have a referral from your primary care physician before seeing a specialist, if you want your treatment and visit to be covered. This is an example of why it's important to have a long-term relationship with your primary care doctor, as they will be able to refer you to a specialist they know and most likely have worked with in the past.

End-of-life professionals

This is a very broad term that encompasses any health care professional or social worker who assists during the last weeks or months of life. An end of life team may include hospital doctors and nurses, a primary care physician, hospice staff, counselors, chaplains, and physical therapists. As an integrative team, they manage pain levels, provide emotional and spiritual support and assist patients and families as they prepare for death. They may also provide guidance about which legal documents need to be signed, such as powers of attorney and health care declarations designed to ensure that the patient's wishes are carried out at the end of their life.

Coping with a terminal illness or imminent death is challenging on a variety of different levels. When you or a loved one faces this scenario, it's important to find a professional that can help you and your family to understand all the decisions that need to be made, especially while you still feel well enough to be involved in the process. It's important to deal with your financial and legal matters as early as possible so that your family isn't left with the burden of trying to interpret your wishes after it's too late to communicate with you.

Pharmacists

Essentially, a pharmacist is a medication expert. They dispense medications to you in accordance to your doctor's prescription. Sometimes they may provide education about how to take the medication. They are also important in detecting incompatibilities between different types of medication. If you have a question about how much medication to take, how often, and what the side effects might be, your pharmacist is an excellent resource.

Medical social workers

Oftentimes when you're faced with a severe medical diagnosis or life-changing injury, every area of your life is affected—from finances to your personal relationships. Many people find themselves completely drowning in details and lists. They have no idea how to cope with all the ways their lives are being transformed. The job of a medical social worker is to help improve the quality of life and the patient's well-being, especially during times of crisis.

Medical social workers may be some of the most underutilized specialists in health care because, so often, people don't want to ask for help. Medical social workers can help patients deal with a multitude of problems in a crisis—everything from comforting you after a devastating diagnosis to assisting you in your search for addiction treatment to helping you navigate your finances when the medical bills start piling up. No matter what challenges you're facing, you do not need go through a crisis alone—a medical social worker can help you.

Physical therapists

This type of health care providers assists you with the challenges of your physical body. They find ways to reduce pain, increase range of motion and mobility, and build muscular strength to lessen stress on your joints. If you've had a musculoskeletal injury, recent surgery, or are having trouble walking or balancing, it's important to get to a physical therapist.

Training and physical therapy is often be your first stop after an injury before considering more serious options such as surgery. These professionals also oversee a critical step after a surgery because a they can—quite literally—help you get back on your feet. Oftentimes, the success or failure of an operation depends on how well you adhere to the physical therapy plan over the long term.

Acupuncturists

A form of Traditional Chinese Medicine (TCM), acupuncture involves having thin needles inserted into your body to improve your Qi, or flow of energy. It might sound terrible, but the needle pricks are relatively pain free. The needles alter the neurohormonal pathways. Acupuncture can be used to treat back pain, headache and a variety of other conditions that may be out of balance.

In the United States, someone can study acupuncture at any school accredited by the Accreditation Commission for Acupuncture and Oriental Medicine (ACAOM). Students going to accredited acupuncture schools must first complete at least two years of study at the baccalaureate level, and many schools require a bachelor's degree. Students in acupuncture programs take courses in Oriental medical theory, diagnosis and treatment techniques, Oriental herbal studies, integrated acupuncture and herbal clinical training, and biomedical clinical sciences. Completing an acupuncture program, graduates have a master's degree, which is the minimum educational requirement to practice in most states.

Massage therapists

Massage therapy is a treatment where the therapist manipulates the muscles in the body to stretch and loosen them as well as to increase blood flow. Numerous studies have shown the value of massage in reducing stress, promoting muscle relaxation and improve mood. A good massage can even help you sleep better.

Licensed massage therapists go through training that focuses on the various muscle groups, joints and spine. The training instills utmost respect for the clients. There are different kinds of massages to help with relaxation such as deep tissue, shiatsu, Swedish, and Thai, among others. A well-trained massage therapist can help you with stiffness, poor physical function and pain. Some encourage you to do meditation during massage for additional benefits.

Nutritionists

As their name suggests, nutritionists can help you achieve optimal health by advising about which foods to eat or avoid and what supplements to take. They can teach you how to read food labels. Nutritionists work in a variety of settings such as cafeterias, hospitals, nursing homes, and schools. Many are also self-employed with their own private practices.

We've all heard the saying that an apple a day keeps the doctor away. As the medical community's understanding of disease continues to grow, doctors and researchers are finding out how incredibly accurate that simple adage really is. In fact, a growing body of research indicates that nutrition plays an important role in the prevention and onset of disease—both minor and major illnesses. For example, doctors now know that diabetes and heart disease can be prevented or greatly reduced through proper nutrition. A nutritionist can help create a plan if you need to reduce your sugar or salt intake or reduce the amount of processed foods or animal products you eat. They can also diagnose whether you're deficient in any critical vitamins or nutrients such as iron, iodine, or calcium.

Herbalists

These specialists use plants (roots, bark, seeds, berries, and flowers) and other natural substances to improve health and prevent and treat illnesses. As herbs and supplements become more popular and their benefits are scientifically documented, the traditional medical community has opened up to herbal remedies. Even some traditional primary care doctors prescribe them. However, depending on where you live and how knowledgeable your doctor is about supplements, it's often a good idea to seek out a specialist.

The supplement and herb business in America is absolutely booming, with over half of Americans taking at least one daily supplement. However, there is very little oversight and regulation of this industry. What this means is that the herb and supplement manufacturers do not have to prove their product is safe the same way pharmaceutical companies do. In fact, the Food and Drug Administration (FDA) does not regulate the supplement industry. Many people assume that just because something comes from a plant or it says "natural" on the bottle that it is completely safe to ingest. This is not the case, and it's absolutely critical to speak to a professional before starting a daily regimen of herbs or supplements. There are also interactions that can occur with more traditional medicines.

Holistic and mindfulness professionals

Much research is being done around the mind-body connection. It has now been scientifically documented that our stress levels and emotional health have a direct impact on our overall physical well-being. Mindful professionals apply the practices of meditation, mindfulness, contemplation, and self-reflection to health.

Mindfulness practices aren't just for gurus and swamis. Scientists have successfully proven the innumerable benefits of a regular meditation. We're discovering that daily meditation can be just as important as a regular cardio workout for health and well-being. If you are interested in incorporating mind-body practices into your daily routine, it's in your best interest to find a professional to help. And no, you don't need to reach nirvana to reap the many rewards.

Clinical Lab Tests

Clinical lab tests are a $73 billion industry in the U.S. alone. It's now routine for doctors to order a wide spectrum of tests as part of the diagnostic process. In the US, it's now possible to request your test results directly from the lab with or without your doctor's consent. However, trying to interpret your own results is not advisable. What may be "normal range" for one person may not be for another based on a variety of factors such as age, sex, race, weight, medications, and medical history. Even something as natural as menstruation can impact test results. Furthermore, you have no basis for understanding how one lab result fits with the information provided by another result. Again, this is when you need a professional eye to look at the whole picture, so be sure to consult with your doctor when assessing your lab results. Here are some of the most common clinical lab tests:

Complete blood count (CBC)

This is a common diagnostic tool for screening your blood. It can help your doctor identify allergies, diagnose infections, and confirm or rule out certain diseases. This exhaustive report provided with the findings of a CBC contains many indicators, but there are typically only three that you need to understand: white count, hemoglobin, and platelets. Everything else on the report is a derivative of these three.

- White blood cells are an indication of your body's immune response. When you have an infection or an allergic reaction, your body will produce more white blood cells. The normal range is 4,300 to 10,800 cells per cubic millimeter.

- Hemoglobin indicates the relative health of your red blood cells. It is a specific protein in the red blood cell that carries oxygen to your organs and tissues. A doctor will look at this indicator to see if your organs are receiving enough oxygen. The normal range is 13 to 18 grams per deciliter for men and 12 to 16 grams per deciliter for women. Low levels can be an indicator for anemia.

- Platelets are the smallest of our blood cells. They are responsible for binding to damaged blood vessels and creating blood clots. Average platelet count is between 150,000 and 450,000 platelets per microliter of blood. Too few platelets mean that you may be at risk for excessive bleeding and could have leukemia, lymphoma, kidney infection, or are on medication. Too many platelets indicate that you may be at risk for blood clots and can also be indicators for diseases such as anemia, cancer, infection, or inflammation. Be sure to tell your doctor if you have a family history of blood clots, strokes, or heart attacks because these types of conditions are related to your platelet count and may be inherited.

Coagulation tests

The CBC is one type of hematology test, but there are several others such as the factor V assay, fibrinogen level, prothrombin time test, thrombin time, and bleeding time. If your doctor suspects that you have a clotting disorder, they may order one of these more specialized tests to measure your blood's ability to clot and how long it takes to clot. Coagulation tests may also be ordered before you go into surgery. Common conditions that cause coagulation problems are hemophilia, thrombophilia, and liver disease. Coagulation tests are generally very safe and side effects such as lightheadedness or soreness at the site are minor.

Basic and comprehensive panels (BMP and CMP)

These tests are related to your metabolism, but not in the narrow way you're used to hearing about metabolism from fad diet books. These tests give a big picture look into the body's chemical processes that use energy. They also test for levels of electrolytes such as calcium, chloride, magnesium, phosphorous, potassium, and sodium to help assess the health of your muscles, the acidity in your blood, and how much water is in your body. The health of your kidneys and liver can also be studied with these tests.

The BMP and CMP may be ordered as part of a routine health exam or during a hospital stay. Doctors will often order a CMP when looking for diabetes or liver or kidney disease. If any results are out of range, more tests are typically ordered to help pinpoint the cause.

Urinalysis (UA)

This is any test that requires a sample of urine. Just like with blood, a lot of information can be obtained by analyzing your urine, especially about the health of your kidneys. This test might be ordered as part of a general yearly screening because it can show evidence of diseases even before you start having symptoms. Your doctor may also order a urinalysis to diagnose certain medical conditions such as kidney stones, urinary infections, diabetes, or kidney inflammation. Urine tests are also common for drug screenings and pregnancy tests.

Because its low cost and simple to perform, a UA is a very common test. It also has a quick turn-around time. It's most often ordered by family health practitioners, internists, obstetricians, gynecologists, and urologists. A macroscopic urinalysis is a visual observation of the urine. Healthy urine is light yellow and clear. Cloudy, dark, or bloody urine may be a sign of infection or disease.

Blood cultures

A blood culture is taken to identify the yeast or bacteria in the blood to determine if there is a systemic infection. This test is usually done when you are showing signs of sepsis such as chills, fever, and rapid heart rate. A blood infection usually starts in one organ of the body such as the urinary tract or the kidneys. If the infection is severe, it will spread to the blood and then the blood carries the infection to other organs causing sepsis. A blood culture can identify the cause so appropriate treatment such as antibiotics can be administered.

Xrays and scans

In addition to blood and urine tests, your doctor may also order machine-assisted tests such as an Xray, computed tomography (CT or CAT) scan, magnetic resonance imaging (MRI) scan or an ultrasound to aid with detection and/or diagnosis. No matter what type of scan you receive, it's important to find out how your doctor interprets that image.

Here are a few great questions to ask about your scan:

- Do you think this scan provides an accurate picture?
- Are there any reasons why this scan might be incorrect?
- What does this scan tell me about my health?
- What are the next steps I should take after this scan?

It's also helpful to have some general knowledge about how each type of scan works and how they are used to detect problems.

Understanding labs, Xrays, CT and MRI Results

An Xray is a black-and-white image of the inside of your body. It's captured using a type of radiation called electromagnetic waves. The amount of radiation that is absorbed impacts how light or dark an area appears on an Xray. Denser materials absorb more radiation and thus appear lighter. For example, bones absorb a lot of radiation, so they show up as white. The air in your lungs absorb very little, so your lungs will appear black. Fat, muscles, and other soft tissues are in the middle and show up as shades of gray.

The most common use of Xrays is to check for broken bones. However, Xrays have many other uses. For example, a chest Xray can spot pneumonia in the lungs or tumors in the breasts. It can also detect an enlarged heart or blocked blood vessels. It is also common to have Xrays taken at the dentist's office. A dental Xray can spot fractures, infections, dental decay, osteoporosis, and bone cancer.

Radiation is toxic to the body, but the amount used in an Xray is very small, about the same amount of radiation you would naturally be exposed to in about ten days. The risk is greatest for small children and fetuses. Always let your doctor know if you might be pregnant because it may be advisable to do an ultrasound instead of an Xray. Routine Xrays have almost zero side effects. Some Xrays, however, require a contrast medium, which may cause reactions in some patients.

A computed tomography or CT scan is a method used for taking pictures of your brain, neck, spine, chest, abdomen, pelvis, and sinuses. Though it is not as detailed as magnetic resonance imaging (MRI), it is still very effective and much quicker and cheaper than an MRI. CTs are often used to identify major problems such as blood inside the skull or fractures.

CTs were derived from the same technology as Xrays. The main difference is that instead of taking only one image, a CT will beam rays around the entire head at different levels to create a series of images. Each image looks like a single 2-dimensional slice of your brain. These image slices start at the top of your head and go to the base of your skull. Just like a traditional Xray, the densest areas will show up lighter on a CT scan. While an Xray is better at examining bones, a CT is preferable when examining soft tissues and organs. A radiologist will review and report on the findings of your CT scan.

Though a CT scan exposes you to a significantly greater amount of radiation than an Xray, the risks associated with a CT scan are still low. Some people may have an allergic reaction to the contrast agent. The odds of a fatal reaction are 1 in 100,000. If an allergic reaction does occur, it will most often happen immediately. There is only a small possibility of a delayed reaction, but if you experience itching or difficulty breathing or swallowing, you should seek medical assistance right away.

Magnetic resonance imaging scans (MRI)

Unlike Xrays and CTs, which use radiation, MRIs use a magnetic field and radio wave energy to take internal pictures of the body. Just like a

CT, an MRI will produce several cross-sectional images like "slices" of a loaf bread. An MRI is very detailed and will often detect abnormalities not visible on any other type of scan. However, MRIs are expensive and time consuming. They last thirty to sixty minutes, so it's typical to have other types of scans done first before an MRI is ordered. For example, if you're experiencing knee pain, an Xray might be ordered first to check the bones. If the bones appear to be normal, then an MRI might be ordered to examine the ligaments.

An MRI is used to scan and detect many abnormalities, but it's commonly used to examine the brain, joints, spine, pelvis, and abdomen. A brain scan is typically used for patients with headaches, blurry vision, hearing loss, and seizures. A spine MRI can locate herniated disks or narrowing of the spinal column. A bone MRI can detect injured ligaments, tendons, bones, muscles, and cartilage.

MRIs are even safer than CTs and Xrays. There is zero risk of radiation, and the contrast dye that is sometimes used is also safer than the dyes for CTs and Xrays. Women who are pregnant are able to get an MRI. Because an MRI uses magnets, it may not be an appropriate scan for patients with metal in their body. A magnetic resonance angiography (MRA) is a specific type of MRI used to examine the blood vessels typically in the neck or brain.

Ultrasounds and Doppler tests

Ultrasounds use sound waves to get internal pictures of your body. The technology is similar to what bats use to navigate in the dark. A sound wave is sent out, when it hits an object, it bounces back as an echo. By measuring the echoes, a computer is able to create an image of your organs. One major benefit of the ultrasound is that the data is being collected in real time, so a doctor can see the blood flowing and the organs moving. It is not a static image like an Xray.

Ultrasounds can be used to monitor a baby in the womb or check for the possible causes of pain, infections, and swelling. Another common use is to help guide the needle during biopsies. You've also probably heard of an echocardiogram or "echo." This is an ultrasound of the heart and is used to diagnose heart conditions such as congestive heart failure.

A Doppler test may also be a part of an ultrasound. It uses a specific technique to monitor blood flow through your arteries and veins. Depending on the type of Doppler test administered, a doctor can determine the speed and direction of the blood flow.

An ultrasound is the safest type of scan, with no known risks. There is also no exposure to radiation since sound waves are being used and no risk of allergic reactions because there is no need for contrast dyes.

Dr. G's Takeaways

- Get recommendations from pharmacists about both lower cost generic medications and what medications covered by your insurance can be substituted at a lower cost.
- If you have to visit a minute clinic or urgent care, bring your medical history.
- More involved procedures such as surgeries will need to be treated in a hospital.
- It's very important to have a primary care physician, even if you're not sick. Building a long-term relationship with your primary care physician increases the likelihood that you will get a correct diagnosis and the best treatment when something goes wrong.
- Almost all insurance plans require you to have a referral from your primary care physician before seeing a specialist, if you want your treatment and visit to be covered.
- Never try to interpret lab results on your own. Always speak to your doctor because he or she will be able to put that result into context and order appropriate follow-up tests.

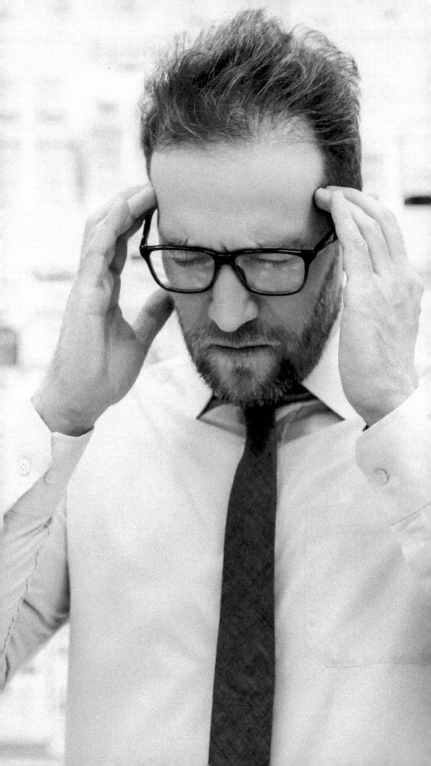

CHAPTER **8**

Tackling Common Health-Care System Headaches

> *"To conquer frustration, one must remain intensely focused on the outcome, not the obstacles."*
>
> T. F. Hodge, From Within I Rise

The number of headaches that my patients report experiencing within the health care system has been increasing over the last few years. They have trouble getting medicines covered by insurance or encounter problems during the prior authorization process that is necessary to have a medicine or test approved. And don't get them started about the difficulty of scheduling appointments with specialists. Everyone struggles with health care costs and insurance coverage restrictions. There are also general accessibility issues that arise from availability, socio-economic inequalities and a person's knowledge about how to navigate the health care system. In this chapter, I will share some tips for overcoming common health care system challenges. My goal is to make things easier for you and empower you with the knowledge you need to receive optimal care as the manager of your own self-health plan.

There can be a good deal of waiting and back-and-forth exchanges that come with securing appointment times and obtaining medications or lab results. These things can be mildly inconvenient at best and filled with complications and stress at worst. Some understanding of the process, along with careful planning, can help you move things along and easily get what you need.

How to make a quick appointment with your doctor

There are two basic considerations that go into scheduling an appointment with your health care provider:

- Availability—both the doctor's and yours
- Urgency—the severity of your symptoms

If you need to see a doctor soon, call as early as possible in the day. The available appointments at a primary care physician's office fill up quickly. If you call for an appointment later in the morning, you're likely to be bumped to the next day. As for *your* availability, you're going to have to be flexible. When weighing whether you can make yourself available when the doctor has an opening, consider what's at stake—your health. Is it worth rescheduling a meeting at work or missing an activity in order to have a doctor diagnose and treat you? If you're calling for an appointment with your health care provider, chances are there's some urgency to your condition, so don't put it off—be flexible and make yourself available.

The urgency of your condition can also influence when you get an appointment. However, the onus falls on you to describe your symptoms and concerns clearly and concisely when you call to make the appointment. It never hurts to take a few minutes to prepare for this call. Write down when your symptoms started, what they are and whether they are getting worse or new symptoms are occurring. Is there a trigger for your symptoms? Have you ever had these symptoms before? Be able to explain what's wrong in a couple of sentences and have your insurance card ready, in case the appointment nurse has questions about your coverage.

If you need to see a health care specialist, getting an appointment requires a different process. Typically, this process begins with your primary-care physician. They make an initial assessment and then refer you to a specialist. In most cases, you won't get in to see a specialist the same day. Often, you have to wait weeks. We'll discuss appointments with specialists in more detail in a few sections.

In both of the above scenarios, your relationship with your doctor can play a role. If you've been with the same medical practice for years, chances are they know you well. Not only is this an advantage because they know your medical history, but the scheduling nurse might try to wiggle you into the schedule because she knows you well. In a practice with multiple doctors, mentioning a specific MD who you've seen in the past may help secure a time slot. This is just another example of the importance of building positive, long-term relationships with your health care providers.

If you can't get the appointment you want, and you need to see a doctor the same day, that's where a medical clinic with walk-in options and longer hours or weekend hours can help. It might not be your first choice, but a clinic can get you the care you need in a pinch. For severe conditions that are potentially life-threatening (e.g., trouble breathing, severe wounds, or poisoning symptoms), skip the doctor altogether and call 911.

How to get your medicines in a timely way

Medical costs aside, getting prescriptions can often be a time hassle. It's not always a straightforward process of just grabbing your medicine off a shelf. There are multiple things that can lead to a delay. On the patient's end, they may have forgotten something like the co-pay, an ID, or their insurance card. Alternatively, limitations to the patient's insurance—for example, the pharmacies it accepts and the prescriptions it covers—can hinder their ability to obtain their prescription. Also, sometimes the prescriber makes a mistake and is the one at fault.

While you can't exactly control other people's mistakes or whether the pharmacy has your medicine in stock, you can make the process easier by remembering to do your part. Look into medicine costs and whether your insurance covers it. Remember to have money for the co-pay along with the correct insurance card and identification. If you were prescribed multiple medicines, be sure to clarify with your doctor about what to expect. Ask questions like:

- What does this drug do?
- How do I use it?
- Anything else I should know?

- What are the drug's side-effects?
- Is adding this drug safe with my other medications?

Not only does this give you an idea of what to look for, it also gives your doctor an opportunity to double-check the prescription they have written for you. You could also ask the pharmacist for information about your medications.

Getting timely lab test results and having them understood by your doctor

The time you spend waiting for lab results while sick may leave you feeling uncertain about what to do. The type of lab tests you take and how urgent your condition is may determine how quickly you get your results back. Lab results taken from the ER have more priority. While common tests involving blood and urine are quickly put through technology, abnormal values may lead to further testing and can take longer. Taking these things into consideration can give you an idea of how long you may have to wait.

If possible, you could try to get the results from the lab directly instead of waiting to see your doctor. When you go in to get tested, ask about results and if it is possible for you to get the results. If asked why, emphasize that you just want to make sure everything is okay and that you want to take care of yourself. It's part of your self-health plan. Depending on the lab, you may be able to find contact information or a way to get your results through their website. A printed copy of the results is ideal. You do have the right to get a copy of your labs, but I highly recommend giving your doctor the opportunity to explain abnormal labs when the lab results are finalized.

But don't just stop there. While the lab report will give you information about your body and your condition, they frequently provide little or no interpretation of the results. Your doctor will also need to interpret your lab results and recommend a course of action based on that interpretation.

How to speed the prior authorization approval process

There are times where your doctor must consult your insurance provider before recommending a treatment. This step ensures that your insurance will cover specific treatments and serves to confirm that you aren't getting unnecessary or duplicate treatments. Nevertheless, some patients may find this process difficult or inconvenient. Here is how to simplify it.

Be sure to talk to the right person. While common sense says call your insurance company, oftentimes this is not the organization responsible for authorizing coverage for your treatments. Many insurance companies outsource such tasks to insurance companies. You may be able to find the correct insurance company by visiting your insurance company's website. If you don't find the information there, contact your insurance provider by phone and ask with whom you should speak.

If possible, do some research and find the insurance company's criteria. This can give you an idea of how to describe your request in the best possible terms to secure coverage and help you understand whether or not they will approve your request. You may need to provide additional details about your health condition to ensure that it meets the requirements for coverage. If your research indicates that your request might not be approved, be sure to make note of the circumstances surrounding that possibility, so that you can address those issues head on, if need be. Let's say, for example, that you have asthma and want a certain inhaler to treat it. However, your insurer requires you to try a preliminary treatment regime before requesting coverage for the alternative treatment that you want, but a severe allergy to something used in that treatment prevented you from doing so. In this case, you would need to explain these unique circumstances to the insurance company in order to secure coverage.

As I've mentioned before, a little preparation can go a long way when you are navigating complex health care systems and processes. Make notes and gather critical information before you make a call to ensure that you can provide detailed and accurate information. Have any notes from recent doctor's visits on hand as well as your insurance information—like how your name is spelled in their database. You want to make sure your submission is clear and is checked for errors. This is especially important since a lot of insurance verification happens via computer. Providing something that is misspelled or incomplete can cause unnecessary delays in securing authorizations.

If for whatever reason you are refused insurance coverage for a procedure, appointment, service or medication, don't give up. See if there is some additional information or action can be completed to meet their coverage guidelines or if there are alternative solutions that your doctor can suggest. The proper ICD 10 codes or diagnostic codes are important when sent to your insurance company and ensure a timely and accurate approval. Get creative and work with your primary care doctor on potential options, if you have a good relationship with him or her.

Appointments with specialists

Let's say that on a cold, dry winter day you wake up with bumpy, red, itchy skin. You're slightly alarmed, because you do not know the cause. You do some online research and wonder if you're having an allergic reaction. Your throat isn't scratchy. You reconsider. Maybe it's just dry skin. Your brain darts from one possibility to the next as you continue your online research. Maybe you are one of the few who develop eczema in their adulthood. Could it be a combination of several medical issues? Baffled and increasingly concerned, you decide to see a dermatologist. You call, but the next available appointment isn't for six weeks. You are left confused and distressed over your skin's appearance and the itchiness.

To compound this problem, your primary health care provider might not have a clear process to refer patients to specialists. In these cases, patients often try to contact specialists directly, leading to appointment "traffic" and delays. Read on to learn about how you could reduce the wait and how to make specific appointments concerning mental health or testing prior to surgery. Here are some tips on how to get an appointment with a specialist in a timely manner:

- Clear communication with your primary care doctor is important. Again, a strong relationship with your primary care doctor can come into play in these situations. Your doctor can evaluate your situation and has the resources to refer you to a suitable specialist, when necessary. He or she can help you find a specialist that meets your needs and preferences. Since your primary provider knows your medical history, they can discuss potential concerns with you and help you understand why an appointment with a specialist might be necessary, or not. Finally, they can make the appointment process more efficient by securing an appointment in a timely fashion and forwarding your health information to the specialist before your appointment.

- The next step requires your input. Sometime before the appointment, call the specialist's office to confirm your appointment and ask whether they have received all necessary information from your doctor. You should also go over your history and information yourself to avoid inconsistencies. If there is an elaborate story of issues and attempted treatments, write it all down and show it to the specialist to ensure that you get the most out of your appointment time.

- Finally, make sure your primary care provider is informed about what happened during your appointment with the specialist. When everyone is on the same page, you can get the treatment you need with less hassle.

Mental health appointments

Like other subspecialties of health, mental health requires the input of a specialist and should be integrated with one's primary health care. That being said, there are unique issues that may accompany mental health care. Some people who need mental health support, don't seek treatment because of the hassle, the cost or concerns about how others may view a mental-health diagnosis or treatment. Today, these concerns are being addressed through innovative new resources and programs. Betterhelp.com is just one example of an online resource where patients can connect virtually with a variety of counselors. However, for the same reasons that I recommend that you build a strong, long-term relationship with your primary health care provider, I also encourage you establish an in-person connection with a counselor in your city or town. You can follow many of the same steps that I suggest in Chapter Five under "Finding the Right Provider" to research and choose your mental health provider.

As with other specialties, securing a mental health appointment may start with talking to your primary physician. Begin the conversation by bringing up your symptoms and how they are impacting your daily life and overall well-being.

An informed and objective opinion from someone who cares about your general health can help you move forward, if you are hesitant or unsure. Additionally, your primary care doctor can guide you as to which type of mental health specialist might be best for you. Insurance coverage for mental health appointments can be trickier, especially in the beginning before you might have a clear diagnosis of your condition. I recommend that you study your coverage early in the process. This can help you budget and plan for treatments, medications, therapies and specialists that might not be covered.

Getting surgical clearance

If need surgery, you might be seen by multiple specialists to prepare. While your physical and medical information should be accessible a week before surgery at the latest, a checkup should be scheduled at least a month in advance. This allows time to discover and treat any conditions that could potentially interfere with your surgery. To prepare for this checkup, jot down what you know about your family's medical history and any complications that may run in your family. For example, a patient whose family has a history of heart attacks may be told to see a cardiologist to get heart tests prior to surgery. The results of the appointment with and tests run by the cardiologist could impact such things as the date of your surgery, the medication used before, during or after your surgery or could even impact how the surgery is performed. Make sure all checkup results are forwarded to the surgeon well in advance of the date of your surgery. This will help prevent delays, should complications be identified.

It is also important to be honest with your surgeon about your lifestyle. Details matter. For example, if you have been taking herbal medications or supplements, your surgeon needs to know. This can prevent potentially dangerous interactions with medications used during the surgery. If you follow a certain diet or exercise regimen, your surgeon needs to know. If you drink or smoke regularly, your surgeon needs to know. Telling your surgeon about any medicines you take is also crucial. You may be advised to stop or change what you are doing in order to be optimally prepared for surgery.

Everyone involved with your surgery—primary care doctors, anesthesiologists, specialists and surgeons—needs to be kept in the loop, so be prepared to answer questions consistently and more than once for different health care providers. Finally, in preparation for your surgery, take care of yourself both physically and emotionally. It will lead to better surgical outcomes.

Dr. G's Takeaways

- Be prepared for appointment scheduling calls by having notes about your symptoms and medical history.
- Know the basics of your insurance coverage and have your member ID, insurance plan, co-pay amount, and your prescription specs ready.
- Talk to the right organization when getting a prior authorization. Sometimes this is an insurance company, not your insurer.
- Use complete, clear and accurate information when applying for coverage and don't give up if you aren't approved.
- Get your primary doctor to refer you to a specialist to lessen wait time.
- Keep an open mind about available mental health resources.
- Depending on the surgical procedure and your health, be prepared to see multiple doctors and answer health history questions starting the month before the surgery.
- If there are multiple doctors involved, make sure to keep everyone in the loop.

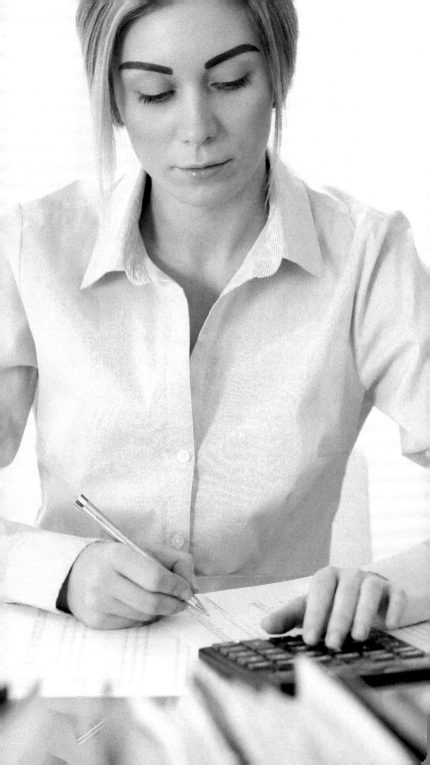

CHAPTER 9

Budgeting for Health-Care Expenses

> *"Unless you control your money, making more won't help, you will just have bigger payments."*
>
> Dave Ramsey, American businessman

People who create a household budget, deal with less stress when paying their bills than those who simply wing it each month. The first group carefully plans and anticipates their monthly expenses and allows for the emergencies and unexpected costs that are part of everyday living. The second group is more likely to run out of money each month. With the skyrocketing cost of health care and the limitations and deductibles of insurance, it is wise to budget for yearly health expenses. Understanding costs and budgeting for health is an important part of any self-health plan.

According to the Kaiser Family Foundation Health Tracking Poll conducted in 2017:

- More than four in ten (43 percent) of adults with health insurance say they have difficulty affording their deductible, and roughly a third say they have trouble affording their premiums and other cost sharing; all shares have increased since 2015.
- About three in ten (29 percent) of Americans report problems paying medical bills, and these problems come with real consequences for some. For example, among those reporting problems paying medical bills, more than seven in ten (73 percent) report cutting back spending on food, clothing, or basic household items.
- Challenges affording care also result in some Americans saying they have delayed or skipped care due to costs in the past year, including 27 percent who say they have put off or postponed getting health care they needed, 23 percent who say they have skipped a recommended medical test or treatment, and 21 percent who say they have not filled a prescription for a medicine.
- Even for those who may not have had difficulty affording care or paying medical bills, there is still a widespread worry about being able to afford needed health care services, with half of the public expressing worry about this.

- Health care-related worries and problems paying for care are particularly prevalent among the uninsured, individuals with lower incomes, and those in poorer health; but women and members of racial minority groups are also more likely than their peers to report these issues.

The study paints a grim picture. Though it may be impossible to budget fully for catastrophic events or chronic illness, it is possible to budget for more predictable health care costs like insurance premiums, deductibles, co-pays, routine and out-of-pocket expenses, uncovered medications, services and providers. It is also possible to create a nest egg of funds for health care surprises.

Determining Your Yearly Health Budget

A great place to start the health care budgeting process is by reviewing how much you spent on health care costs last year. If you have not reviewed your health care costs in a few years, you might be shocked when you find out just how much you have been spending. If you can't gather the information to come up with last year's health care spending, then it's time to start organizing your health care paperwork and collecting this data, perhaps in a spreadsheet.

Don't make the mistake of underestimating costs when it comes to health care expenses. Americans pay nearly $3.4 trillion dollars a year (yes, that's *trillion!*) for health care...and costs just keep rising. With this in mind, it's always better to budget for a higher dollar figure. This way, you can be pleasantly surprised if the actual cost turns out to be lower than what you had anticipated. Here's a simple guide to help you start keeping track of your health expenses and begin to plan a budget for them:

Monthly insurance premium	$ _____
Out-of-pocket maximum payments for emergencies	$ _____
Copay costs for routine doctor visits	$ _____
Costs for prescriptions and over-the-counter medicines	$ _____
Other medical costs (e.g. contacts, eye glasses, dental appointments)	$ _____
Well-being and preventative costs (e.g. yoga classes, gym membership)	$ _____

Add up these expenses to get your annual budget and then break this cost down to the amount of money you'll need monthly to cover these expenses. That's what simple health care budget looks like. But there's one more addition to your budget that we need to explore, so let's move on to the next section.

Start an Emergency Health Fund

In addition to a budget to cover your health care basics, you need to save something each month for potential major medical emergencies—those unexpected events that life can throw us like a car accident or unexpected injury or major illness. Even if you're an optimist, it's just not smart to risk your financial future because you haven't saved for medical surprises. According to a Kaiser Family Foundation study in 2014, called "Medical Debt Among People with Health Insurance":

Medical debt can affect almost anyone. People we interviewed ranged in age from 20s to 60s and lived in various states. Some were single, others headed families. Their annual incomes ranged from less than $10,000 to more than $100,000. Most were insured continuously in job-based group plans; a few were covered in non-group policies. Two others were insured at the outset of illness, and then lost coverage. Three were uninsured the entire time. For most in our study, this instance of medical debt was the first time they had experienced serious financial or credit problems. The onset of an illness, accident, or pregnancy generated expenses that they did not anticipate and which they were unprepared to pay. Some faced tens of thousands of dollars in medical debt. For others, just a few thousand dollars of bills proved unaffordable, particularly when a chronic illness meant bills would continue year after year.

Like it or not, it's smart to start an emergency health fund. Ask yourself how much you can put away each month for your emergency health fund. It is entirely up to you. Some people like to put away a standard ten percent of their income. My advice is to put away more, if you can afford it. Do the math and begin to build an emergency health fund that you can afford, but that will create the safety net you'll need in a time of crisis.

- Research shows that households with emergency savings below $500 are more prone to worry, loss of sleep and other ill effects. Set a goal to save at least $500 for emergencies.
- Once you have $500 saved, congratulate yourself for your good work and then set a goal to save enough money to cover at least one month of your financial obligations should an emergency force you to take a leave of absence at work and perhaps not get paid.
- Set up an automated transfer into savings from your checking account once a month to move the money you've designated into your emergency account.
- Use a savings app or financial product that automatically saves every time you make a

purchase. For example, some apps will round up to the nearest dollar of every purchase and put the remaining change into savings. In other words, if your purchase is $3.55, the savings app would add $0.45 to your account. This small savings will add up over time.

Keep Track of Health Expenses

Tracking your health costs doesn't have to be fancy or complicated. You can use a basic spreadsheet or simple budging websites or apps. But to have an informed budget, you'll need to keep track of your bills, subscriptions, invoices and other important paperwork and files. It may seem like you are drowning in bureaucratic health care information at times, but rest assured, having that information at your fingertips when you need it is a good thing. Find a safe place to organize and store all of these records in one place. This will make them easy to locate and access when you need them.

The American Association of Retired Persons (AARP) offers the following tips on what types of information you should save and file:

- Copies of bills from doctors/clinics/hospitals
- Anything written from your insurance com-

pany, including your Explanation of Benefits (EOB)
- Notes from conversations with your insurance company or your doctor about billing and payments
- Payment records/receipts
- Copies of any referral forms
- Insurance premium information
- Transportation expense records

It requires some discipline and time, however organizing your medical paperwork and keeping a close eye on your medical expenses could save you a lot of money in the long run.

Saving on Medications

Your prescription medicine may come with a new side effect: financial pain. Like health care in general, prescription-drug costs continue to skyrocket, according to the Centers for Medicare & Medicaid Services. The sickest Americans bear the biggest burden. Some 43 percent of those in fair or poor health say it's somewhat or very difficult to afford their medications, and 37 percent say they've skipped out on filling a prescription because of cost, according to the Kaiser Family Foundation.

What has changed? Generic drugs—long an affordable alternative to name-brand medicines—

have now become part of the problem. The average price of the fifty most popular generic drugs has increased 373 percent in a recent five-year period, according to OptumRx, a pharmacy insurance company. One culprit is consolidation: after a decade of mergers, three big companies now control 40 percent of the generics market, says Gerard Anderson, professor at the Johns Hopkins Bloomberg School of Public Health. Weaker competition means drug companies can charge your insurer more. Meanwhile, pricey new miracle drugs—like hepatitis C treatment Sovaldi ($1,000 per pill for an 84-pill course)—are also a key factor in forcing up overall medication costs.

If you have a good health insurance plan, here are some tips to help you save money on your medications:

- Use generic brands whenever possible. However, all generic drugs are not created equal, so ask your physician to guide and advise you. He or she will know if a generic brand is available and will work for your particular health condition.
- Order your prescriptions by mail. On average, a consumer can save nearly 30 to 40 percent on the costs associated with many common medications.
- Many health care plans now suggest (some even require) that their members use a certain

drugstore. Often, they've negotiated special pricing. Do your homework on these offers to find out if they offer better prices than the drugstore you are currently using.

If you find yourself without health insurance, or are going through some difficult financial struggles, do not let that stop you from getting the medications you need. Here are some ideas on how to save on medications, if you are not insured:

- Ask your physician for sample medications. Most physicians will have a supply of samples from their pharmaceutical reps on hand. Explain your situation and ask for the medications you need.

- Shop around for a discount pharmacy. Competition is fierce for your medication dollars, with the popular chain drugstores in nearly every neighborhood these days. Don't hesitate to shop around for the best prices. Places like Walmart and Target are likely to be less expensive than a Walgreens or a Rite Aid. Also check with supermarkets that have a pharmacy. Most of them also offer a reduced price for many common prescription drugs, some even offer certain medications for free.

- Check with pharmaceutical companies and websites. Many have patient-assistance programs to aid people who have a hard time affording their treatment. There may be income limits and other requirements, but it's worth researching. Check <u>RxAssist.org</u>, <u>patientadvocate.org</u>, and <u>pparx.org</u> to find programs for your medications.

Strategies to Save on Costly Health Tests and Procedures

Health tests and procedures can literally save your life, so if your physician or health care provider says it is time to have something done, don't put it off because of the cost. Of course, if you a mediocre health insurance plan, or no plan at all, then knowing that you need a medical procedure can certainly cause stress. These are the types of situations where your health care budget and savings can be used.

Even though fully-covered tests are getting more common, most still require copays and sometimes you have to shoulder the full cost, if you haven't reached your insurance deductible. Be creative and look for ways to save on every test you take. Prices can vary widely for the same test. Putting these strategies into action can help you lower costs and keep more money in your pocket.

• Choose professionals and institutions that are transparent about their costs. Start by checking your health insurer's website—many list doctors that insurers believe offer quality care at fair prices. Keep in mind that MRIs, CT scans, and other imaging tests often cost much less at free- standing radiology centers (rather than hospitals). Just be sure the facility is accredited by the American College of Radiology and that your doctor will accept the results. And when your doctor orders a blood test, ask about all your options.

- Discuss the urgency, risks and benefits of each test and procedure with your doctor. Far too often patients leave the doctor's office and have no idea why they are having a test done. Your doctor is on your side when it comes to keeping you healthy and helping you get well if you are sick. They will be honest with you about the urgency of having a test done if you let them know you may have financial or insurance issues.

- Compare prices for procedures ranging from knee surgeries to vasectomies. This can help eliminate most of the surprise bills that show up long after their wounds have healed. Amino, a health data company is already helping connect patients to doctors in their areas based on quality data. The new tool greatly expands its pricing data and covers about 550,000 physicians, 49 procedures and 129 insurance companies.

There are some other websites that will help you compare prices for medical procedures. Take some time and explore these:

- Healthcare Bluebook (www.healthcareblue-book.com) has a simple platform where you compare providers by quality and cost. You select the type of care or medication you need and enter your zip code into the Fair Price search tool. Then an average fee based on your location pops up. Once you receive the estimate, you can use it while shopping to ensure the amount you pay for a procedure or medication is fair.

- At Save On Medical (www.saveonmedical.com) you can look up costs for procedures like mammograms, Xrays or ultrasounds. The search process at Save On Medical is very similar to the process at Health care Blue Book. You enter your location and your medical procedure to get a list of providers in your area, along with pricing info. You can also set up appointments through the site and pay in advance to lock in discounted rates.

- The FAIR Health site (www.fairhealthcon-sumer.org) aims to bring transparency to health care costs and health insurance with informative articles and a medical cost estimator search bar. One of its many resources is the Health Insurance 101 page which explains insurance in layman's terms. To use the search tool you enter your location, whether you're insured or not, and the type of procedure you need. Keep in mind, you can only perform up to ten searches per week on the FAIR Health site, so search wisely.

Health Savings Accounts (HSA)

A health savings account allows you to set aside money on a pre-tax basis to pay for qualified medical expenses. This type of account can be used only if you have a High Deductible Health Plan (HDHP). High-deductible plans usually have lower monthly premiums than plans with lower deductibles. By using the untaxed funds in an HSA to pay for expenses before you reach your deductible and other out-of-pocket costs like copayments, you reduce your overall health care costs. HSA funds roll over year to year if you don't spend them. Also, HSAs may earn interest.

Funds you withdraw from your HSA are tax-free when used to pay for qualified medical expenses. The expenses must be primarily to alleviate or prevent a physical or mental defect or illness, including dental and vision. A list of these expenses is available on the IRS website, www.irs.gov in IRS Publication 502, "Medical and Dental Expenses."

Any funds you withdraw for non-qualified medical expenses will be taxed at your income tax rate plus 20 percent tax penalty if you're under 65.

Here are some examples of eligible medical expenses:

- Eye exams or eye surgery
- Prescription drugs
- Mental health therapy
- Lab fees
- Dental treatments
- Weight loss programs

Here are some examples of ineligible medical expenses:

- Hair transplants
- Funeral expenses
- Nutritional supplements
- Insurance premiums
- Maternity clothes
- Nonprescription drugs

Everyone knows how important accurate reporting on your income tax returns is. And when you have a health savings account, there are a few extra forms that you will need to file with your tax return. Remember, the IRS may modify its list of eligible expenses from time to time. As always, consult your tax advisor should you require specific tax advice.

Here is a link to the information that pertains to HSAs with official forms that need to be filed:

https://www.1040.com/tax-guide/health-and-life-insurance/hsas-and-your-tax-return/

Health Reimbursement Account (HRA)

Health Reimbursement Account. An employer-funded health benefit plan where the employer reimburses employees for out-of-pocket medical expenses and insurance premiums.

Flexible Savings Account (FSA)

A Flexible Savings account is available to anyone without an HSA. An FSA is similar to an HSA in that it is funded by pretax dollars for qualifying expenses. The contribution cap is smaller than an HSA and the money cannot be rolled over from year to year. A limited purpose FSA can be set up in conjunction with an HSA to cover expenses such as dental or vision.

There's an App for That

Just about everything on the planet has an app associated with it, and Health Savings Accounts are no different. A quick Google search will help you locate a variety of apps.

Here is a Website that lists some of the top HSA apps: http://appcrawlr.com/android-apps/best-apps-hsa-account

Organization and financial planning is a key component of any successful self-health plan. You'll experience less anxiety if you organize your medical paperwork, assess your current health spending, create a health care budget and set aside a portion of your income in a medical emergency fund.

Dr. G's Takeaways

- Don't put off needed treatment because of cost. It could have undesirable consequences.
- Create an annual health budget with at least these three main items: your insurance premium, routine out-of-pocket expenses and medication expenses. The more granular you can be about the items in your budget, the more useful it will be to you.
- To determine your yearly budget, use how much you spent the year before
- Start an emergency health fund and transfer a set amount every month.
- Track your expenses using online programs, spreadsheets, or apps.
- Save on medications, by asking your doctor for free samples or shopping at a discount or insurer-preferred pharmacy.
- Before committing, have a heart-to-heart talk with your doctor regarding whether you really need a specific test or procedure.

- Choose professionals and institutions that are transparent about the cost of labs, diagnostic procedures and surgical procedures.
- Set up a health savings account to pay for qualified medical expenses and save on your taxes

MEDICAL INSURANCE

HEALTH INSURANC

months (2 years), have you used any tobacco product?

ast regular check-up with a physician more than **18 months ago**?

ast 12 months, have you used or been prescribed home oxygen for any medical condition?

ve you ever had 2 of the following **3 conditions**
diabetes • stroke • **ANY heart condition**
Note: for the purposes of this Medical Questionnaire, **ever had** means you have been diagnosed, bee
medication, or taken prescription medication for the condition.

Was your **FIRST** heart bypass surgery **MORE** than 10 years ago? or your first procedure was **less than 10 ye**
Note: If you have **never** had heart bypass surgery OR your first procedure was **less than 10 ye**

For questions 6 to 10, in order to score 0, you must CORRECTLY answer NO to all parts of the que

For ANY heart condition, have you EVER:
a) been diagnosed with **ANY heart condition**?
b) been prescribed medication for **ANY heart condition**?

CHAPTER **10**

Navigating Insurance

> *"I may not have gone where I intended to go, but I think I have ended up where I needed to be."*
>
> Douglas Adams, *The Long Dark Tea-Time of the Soul*

I've been in private medical practice since 2001. From the beginning, I wanted to serve all my near north side Chicago neighborhood, so I accepted most all private insurance, public aid and Medicare. When the Affordable Care Act came into being, I accepted those plans as well. Patients regularly share the frustration they encounter when they have to deal with their insurance companies. They tell me how they don't understand their policies or know what's in and out of network. Because I work with so many insurance plans, I have been able to provide advice when my patients struggle to get needed medications, services or tests. I know it's not a fun topic, but it's an important one. You can't take control of your health care if you don't understand insurance. Again, having the right insurance to fit your needs is an important component of your self-health plan.

I regularly feel my patients' pain in dealing insurance company policies and procedures. My office manager keeps a binder of the twenty insurance plans my practice accepts in the front office. It demonstrates the labyrinth that insurance has become. In our dealings with insurance companies, we notice big differences in how each handle prior authorizations, procedure and medication coverage, and other health care services and programs. Sometimes there's even variability on these things *within* the same insurance company! We also notice that policies change frequently, adding to the confusion. We work hard for our patients, trying to find easier and more expedient ways to take care of such things as prior authorization, coverage and reimbursement. The time spent to get what I need for my patients from insurance companies has increased three-fold since I started my practice. I want to pass on what we have learned from these daily struggles.

With skyrocketing costs and growing complexity, the insurance industry needs to be reformed. I know I'm not alone in this belief as my patients share this sentiment frequently with me. The insurance needs to standardize, simplify and streamline many policies and processes. There needs to be more transparency and fairness in the industry's policies. I often think of what I could do with all the time we would save if we didn't have such a heavy and time-consuming administrative burden when it comes to insurance providers. All those frustrating phone calls could be replaced by seeing more patients and providing more health care education. While we wait for change, though, you'll benefit from some insider tips. In the coming sections, I will show you how to select an insurance company and policy and then maximize your plan. I'll also show you how to switch to a new policy, if you're not happy with your current one. Let's dive in.

Terminology of Health Care Coverage

It is important that you take the time to understand the meanings of all the acronyms, abbreviations and long strings of letters that dot your plan descriptions. Unraveling the alphabet of insurance-speak is the start of being able to invest in practical research. This will help you make more well-informed decisions regarding your health care plan. Nearly every plan requires three payments from the consumer, which vary in cost and the charge for one impacts the cost for the other. Below are common acronyms, terminology and jargon used by insurance companies.

Co-pay

The amount of money you owe for a doctor's visit. It could be 80/20, with your insurance paying eighty percent of the visit or procedure and you paying twenty percent Your co-pay can also be a flat amount and can vary if you go out of network.

Coverage

This term refers to those health care services that are "covered." This means that your insurance company will pick up a portion or the entire cost of health care visit or service. Your coverage can vary widely depending on the health insurance plan you have.

Deductible

The annual amount of money that you must pay before your insurance kicks in. It is also referred to as an "out of pocket maximum." A higher deductible means lower monthly premiums and a lower deductible means higher monthly premiums. Depending on your plan, a high deductible may be as much as $5,000 per year or more per family member, but your premiums will be lower, if you opt for a high-deductible plan.

EOB

Explanation of Benefits

HDHP

High Deductible Health Plan

In-network

Working with doctors who are within your insurer's network of providers. In-network providers may want to send you to an out-of-network specialist, lab or hospital facility. Always determine whether there is an alternative provider who is in your insurer's network. Otherwise, you could be looking at a higher co-payment and other out-of-pocket expenses.

Open Enrollment

Refers to the annual period of time in which someone may sign up for or make changes to his or her policy. The exception to open enrollment is marriage or the birth of a child, which can be done at any time.

Out-of-Network

Availing facilities that are out of the range of your choice of doctors. You often have to pay higher copays and out-of-pocket expenses for a health care provider who is out-of-network.

Out-of-pocket expenses

The amount of money you pay until you hit a co-payment cap or deductible, after which your insurance kicks in and starts paying in full.

Premium

The monthly fee you pay to your insurance company. Your premium will be less if you are single, more if you are married, and even more if you include children in your plan. If you are employed, your employer will probably be paying a partial amount of your premium.

Understanding Your Insurance Options

Further adding to the complexity of choosing a plan, are a bewildering number of different types of coverage. Let's take a closer look at each:

Employer-based insurance

The majority of Americans receive their health insurance through their employers. Employers generally pay a portion of their employee's monthly premiums and, because they purchase in bulk, insurance costs are often lower. Some businesses and corporations offer rich wellness programs along with Fitbits or onsite massage. These employers may also offer a variety of insurance package levels ranging from bronze to gold. They may also offer an HMO (Health Maintenance Organization option) and a PPO (preferred provider), and you will be required to choose.

It is best to meet with an HR representative and have him or her review the benefits included in each level and the costs of the premiums and co-pays.

Smaller employers may offer one coverage option only. It is still critical to read through the plan. If you believe that the offered plan does not meet government standards, you can compare your company's insurance plan to the Affordable Care Act exchanges in your state. These plans are often confusing, with people buying high deductible plans to lower their premiums and opting for services they may not need. For more information, visit https://www.healthcare.gov/quick-guide/one-page-guide-to-the-marketplace.

Some companies and businesses are self-insured, meaning they bypass a third-party administrator. When these companies crunched their numbers, they found it more cost effective to pay for each occurrence out of pocket. They do not pay a fixed premium to an insurance company. There are, of course, tax and cash flow benefits to a company that are not subject to state regulations.

Self-Insured group plans typically require that employees pay premiums. These premiums are held by the company rather than turned over to an insurance company. Self-insured plans must still abide by all applicable federal laws, including: the Employee Retirement Income Security Act (ERISA); Health Insurance Portability and Accountability Act (HIPAA); Consolidated Omnibus Budget Reconciliation Act (COBRA); the Americans with Disabilities Act (ADA); the Pregnancy Discrimination Act; the Age Discrimination in Employment Act; the Civil Rights Act; and various budget reconciliation acts such as Tax Equity and Fiscal Responsibility Act (TEFRA), Deficit Reduction Act (DEFRA), and Economic Recovery Tax Act (ERTA).

Health care sharing plans

These plans are faith-based, in general, but some of them are open to anyone. In these plans, members share the medical expenses. The way it works is fairly simple: everyone pays a certain amount each month and then a yearly premium.

Health Maintenance Organization (HMO)

This stands for Health Maintenance Organization. Provides financing and care for doctors and hospital stays for a monthly fee. There is no co-pay.

There are lower out-of-pocket expenses and either low or no deductibles. There is a strong focus on preventative care. Membership may include wellness programs and gym memberships. You are assigned to a primary care doctor who must approve all your visits to a specialist. You are limited to certain participating doctors and hospitals in the HMO network.

Medicare

Open to all adults over age 65 and individuals with disabilities, Medicare is a federal health insurance program that requires a monthly payment based on income. The program offers several types of insurance. To learn more visit https://www.medicare.gov/. Many seniors enrolled in Medicare also opt to purchase supplemental health insurance to cover deductibles, premiums and other expenses not covered by Medicare. The AARP is a good place to begin exploring supplemental insurance plans.

Medicaid

Medicaid provides health coverage to eligible low-income adults, children, pregnant women, elderly adults and people with disabilities. It is funded by the federal government and administered by the states, according to federal requirements. As of February 2018, there were 68 million people covered by Medicaid. For more information about Medicaid visit https://www.medicaid.gov/

Point of Service (POS)

Point of Service is a type of managed care plan that is lower cost than a PPO, but choices are more limited. You are still assigned a primary care physician, but you can be referred to specialists outside the network.

Preferred Provider Organization (PPO)

Preferred Provider Organization. If you are a person who wants a choice of doctors and care providers, you will want to consider a PPO. PPOs are care providers and hospitals that operate within a network. Premiums and co-pays are higher. There are deductibles to meet, and sometimes you may have to pay the provider directly and wait for reimbursement. If you go out of network, a portion of that service will not be covered. Sometimes there are tiers of coverage for out of network providers.

Private individual insurance

If you are self-employed, own a small company, or find yourself without insurance, you will need to explore options for private insurance. Large employers offer group memberships, meaning the costs are lower due to volume. Individuals and small companies do not have the buying power of a large corporation and consequently wind up paying significantly higher premiums as well as higher deductibles when purchasing directly through an insurance company. Keep in mind that as a small business, your copayments, deductibles and premiums may be tax deductible.

Health shares are not an insurance policy, so the rules of the game are different. The benefit is that share plan costs are lower, but their coverage can be limited. Care sharing plans may not pay for a preexisting condition at the outset, but later on, depending on the share plan, it might be included. Psychiatric counseling, for instance, may not be a reimbursable service.

Unlike insurance companies, you have the option to see any doctor you choose. Four major health care sharing plans are as follows: Samaritan, Liberty Health care, Medi-Share | Christian Care Ministry. You can learn more about this type of health care coverage here: http://www. medicalcostshare.com/comparison-of-major-health care-sharing-ministries.html

Veterans' Health Care

Available to those who served in the United States Armed Forces. Coverage from the Veteran's Affairs Administrations (VA) can be used in conjunction with private coverage.

Researching and Evaluating Insurance Plans

Most of us would rather do almost anything besides comb through the fine print of a health-insurance contract. Dull as it may seem, underestimating the coverage you may need for yourself or your family can result in some dire financial and health consequences—like receiving expensive bills for services you assumed were covered. My advice is to be fully informed about your insurance plan. Treat your insurance plan like your financial portfolio and give it the attention it deserves. As they say, the devil is in the details, so carve out the time, pour some coffee and dig in. Your financial well-being—not to mention your life—may depend on it.

Over the years, my patients have shared how they have researched their insurance plans. I've seen them change plans. I've watched them identify surprising loopholes and confront unwarranted red tape. In this chapter, I've combined my experience as a doctor navigating health insurance from the practitioner side of things and my patients' insights from the consumer side. Hopefully, combining our hard-earned wisdom can make your health plan selection easier by helping you focus on the most important considerations. Here are some of the topics we'll cover:

- Assessing what you need in a medical plan
- Understanding your insurance options
- Using the government health insurance exchanges
- Defining important health care coverage terminology
- Understanding your policy and putting it all together

To effectively evaluate a health care plan, you must first evaluate yourself. Begin, by answering the following questions:

- How old are you?
- Are you single or married?
- What is your gender?
- Are you planning to have children?
- Do you have children? How old are they?
- Do you need vision care?
- Will your spouse be included in your plan?
- How old is he or she?
- What is the state of your health?
- Your spouse's health?
- The health of your children?
- Are you a veteran?
- Is your spouse a veteran?
- What are your particular concerns?
- Are you or anyone in your family on a specific medication?
- Do you or anyone in your family have a chronic medical condition?

- Do you or anyone in your family have a familial history of a debilitating or even mildly debilitating disease?
- Does anyone have an addiction challenge?
- Will you need vision care?
- Will anyone need braces?
- Are you serious about preventative care?
- Do you have pre-existing conditions?
- What is your budget for insurance?

Insurance needs are very personal

Tracey just turned 27 years old. She is single and in good health. This is the first year she will be enrolling in her employer's health insurance plan. Since Tracey has no preexisting conditions, is not planning on starting a family, and is concerned only with wellness visits, a flu shot, an annual pap smear and birth control prescription, she would be a good candidate for a high-deductible plan. She might also want to think about contributing to a flexible savings account.

Gavin is 50 years old, married with three children, and a graphic artist at an advertising agency. He and his wife will need more preventative and wellness care than Tracey, including colonoscopies, mammograms and continued care for their youngest daughter who has scoliosis. Gavin's son needs braces, but they are not covered under his plan. Contributions to an HSA (Health Savings Account) can help him pay the orthodontist.

Even with a quick look at these two scenarios, it quickly becomes apparent that everyone has different insurance needs. Age, marital status, health status, chronic conditions, gender—all of these are factors in choosing the best insurance policy for your needs.

Marital status and family considerations

Your marital and family status plays an important role in evaluating insurance options. If you are married and you and your spouse both carry insurance, you will have three, or possibly four, options:

- Dual plans. You each carry separate insurance. If there are children, you put them on either your or your spouse's plan. This can be very expensive. You will need to meet two deductibles and pay two premiums. Two plans do not provide double coverage.
- You select the best plan for your family. Some companies charge a "spouse surcharge," if your spouse decides to join your company plan.
- If neither of the above options work, you can purchase your own insurance.

- Depending on your employer and the state in which you live, you may be able to coordinate your benefits using one plan to pay for key coverage and the other to cover other accrued expenses.

If you have a domestic partner, there are different considerations. Some company health plans allow you to add a domestic partner. Check with your plan administrator to see if this is possible. You may have to provide proof of cohabitation and shared expenses. If both of you have insurance coverage, make sure to understand the full benefits of each of your plans. One plan may be better than the other for your specific needs. For example, if your plan doesn't cover chiropractic, but your partner's plan does, then you may want to go with your partner's plan, if that type of coverage is important to you.

For those of you who have a child going to college, don't automatically opt in to the college or university's health plan for your student. Instead, compare the costs of purchasing health coverage for the child through their college to the cost of keeping your child on your family plan. You might be surprised by what you find.

If you feel you will be leaving your job in the near future, use the money in your FSA (Flexible Savings Account) whenever possible, otherwise the money will revert to your employer. You'll find a list of all FSA-covered deductibles at www.irs.gov/publications//p502. Consider opening an HSA (Health Savings Account). The tax scenario is more favorable for an FSA, but HSA offers peace of mind as it is portable from job to job. COBRA and Medicare premiums can be paid through an HSA account. An HSA account is portable and can be opened even if you don't have a job. Both HSA and FSA accounts are funded with pretax dollars. Check with your accountant to determine which option is best for you.

Evaluating Your Plan: Is Your Insurance Right for You?

If you are still enrolled in the same high deductible insurance plan you had when you were a 28-year-old single and you are now the 37-year-old parent of six-year-old twins, I'm pretty sure that I can say with confidence that your insurance plan probably isn't working very well for you these days. It's time to reassess. Here are is a sampling of some questions you might ask yourself as you consider changing insurers or policies:

- What aspects of my health care are absolutely essential?
- Does it pay to lower my deductible but raise my premiums?
- Do I have the cash flow to contribute to an HSA or FSA to help pay my deductibles?

- Will I need fertility treatment in the future?
- Will my teenager still need physical therapy?
- Will I decide to retire this year?

Use the following calculation to determine what your out-of-pocket medical expenses were the previous year and what they are likely to be this year.

Deductible + Co-payment for medical visits and prescriptions
+ Monthly Premium (x12)
- Minus Tax Benefits (if any)
= Total Spent

Use this worksheet to create a comparison between last year's and this year's potential changes to your plan.

Last Year	Expense	This Year	Average Cost

Completing this worksheet should give a good overview of what's ahead and help you plan for those expenses. This exercise might also help you decide if it's time to switch to a new plan.

When it is time to either select a new plan or re-enroll in your existing plan for a new year, make sure that you are completely satisfied with all aspects of the health insurance company. Factor in the monthly premiums, your deductibles, what is covered versus what's not covered, and so on. If keeping the same physician is important to you and your family, make sure they are a part of the plan's network. Many people switch plans just to keep their physician. In the end, it's a personal choice.

Using a broker to find health insurance

All United States citizens are eligible to purchase private insurance. Even someone on Medicare can buy private supplemental insurance. Some people find it helpful to use a health insurance agent or broker. Because brokers work with a variety of insurance companies, they tend to have a broader understanding of companies' offerings and key benefits. They are commission-based, which is a double-edged sword. They may be more motivated to earn your business year after year by getting you the best deal possible, or they may try to sell you a policy with unnecessary bells and whistles since that would earn them a higher commission. The best way to nail down the best deal possible is the annual review and re-shopping of coverage. The best way to avoid unnecessary "bells and whistles" is to remember that your needs guide what you purchase. If you don't need "bells and whistles", don't purchase them.

Using the government exchanges to find Insurance

Presently, insurance under the Affordable Care Act (ACA)—also known as "Obamacare"—can be purchased through online health insurance marketplaces or exchanges. The insurance is offered through state or federal governments, or a partnership between them. It was designed to offer coverage to all.

If you are not comfortable with or cannot afford the insurance your employer is offering, you may be able to purchase insurance through one of the health insurance exchanges, which offer four tiers of coverage: bronze, silver, gold and platinum. The brighter the "metal," the greater the coverage and the more expensive the plan. You may qualify for subsidies for premiums or deductibles or both if your income is $12,000 or less for individuals.

Navigators are available to assist you with enrolling in an exchange health plan. Navigators are trained to answer questions, provide details regarding the exchange plans, and to assist if a claim is rejected. However, they cannot make recommendations. They are paid through a grant. Healthcare.gov can direct you to a navigator in your area or someone who is certified to advise you on insurance matters.

Also available are certified application counselors who are not required to perform outreach. They may work through a nonprofit organization and, similar to navigators, they can explain each plan to you but cannot tell you which program to select. Insurance brokers can also enroll you in an exchange plan and help guide your decision. Keep in mind that your insurance broker may receive a commission for selling you a particular plan. Establishing a health insurance usage plan during open enrollment can ultimately help you save money and determine if your current plan is right for you.

Although a lot of uncertainty has been introduced into this option under the Trump administration, for now preexisting conditions cannot be excluded, and there is a focus on paid wellness visits. The law also lifts the lifetime cap of covered occurrences to $1 million. Participating insurers must meet ten criteria, or the ten essential benefits, including coverage for mental health, addiction, and chronic disease. The ten essential health benefits mean there can be no contributing fees to these services in small group plans. The required benefits are:

- Ambulatory services—outpatient care
- Emergency room services
- Hospitalization—inpatient care
- Maternity and newborn care
- Mental health, substance abuse and behavior health treatment
- Prescription drugs
- Rehabilitative services and devices
- Laboratory services
- Preventative, wellness and management of chronic diseases
- Pediatric services including dental and vision services

Employers of 50 or more individuals, or employers with self-funded plans are exempt from offering the ten essential health benefits. If they choose to offer them, there cannot be a lifetime limit of coverage. Note that plans for large corporations and smaller companies will differ.

Understanding Your Policy

The key to comprehending 21st century insurance plans is to understand the various nuances underpinning the Affordable Care Act and the plans that are offered on the federal and state exchanges. This will give you an idea of what you can expect from a private plan or a plan offered by your employer. Once you know the basics, then you can make good decisions regarding your choices.

It's very important to understand the details around how your insurer handles in-network versus out-of-network expenses. If you don't, the mistakes can be quite costly. Take, for example, Ashley and David who were relieved to learn that their health insurance plan would cover up to twenty visits with a speech therapist for their six-year-old daughter who had been diagnosed with a mild speech disorder. They started taking their daughter to a speech pathologist who charged $80 for each session. They were told that they had to pay this amount until the met their $1,500 annual deductible. Once Ashley and David reached their deductible, they expected that their daughter's speech therapy sessions would continue and finally be covered for the twenty visits allowed in their plan. They faced a rude surprise when they were told by their insurer that there would be no reimbursement for future speech therapy sessions. The reason? They'd already reached the maximum number of twenty sessions while working toward their deductible. Had Ashley and David understood this from the outset, perhaps they would have paid for a less expensive speech pathologist or met their deductible with other expenses first.

The language found in most insurance policies can be quite tricky, so read your policy closely and ask for advice and clarification whenever you're not sure.

Your primary care doctor can be a great resource in this regard. Not only has he or she probably seen it all when it comes to coverage surprises, but your primary care doctor can help guide you, plan to meet with him or her at the end of the year to determine what tests, lab work and procedures will be required for you in the upcoming year. If you do not have a primary care doctor, you might want to talk to a navigator about what your insurance needs might be for the year. Remember, navigators are individuals or organizations that are trained to help you look for health coverage options through the government's health care marketplace, including completing eligibility and enrollment forms. These individuals and organizations are required to be unbiased.

How to Maximize Your Coverage

If you take the time to learn the ropes of your insurance, you'll be surprised by how much time and money you can save. Below are several ways to get the most out of your health insurance plan:

- If medically possible, leave major medical procedures until the end of the year when you have met or almost fully met your deductibles and your total out of pocket expenses. This will save you having to pay out a big cash outlay at one time.
- If lowering the cost of health insurance is a priority for you, join an HMO over a PPO. HMOs are usually significantly less expensive. You will, however, have a much more limited choice of providers and services.
- If you have a high deductible plan, it pays to shop around for service providers. For instance, eye exams may vary in price and you can choose a less-expensive provider.
- Try to stay in-network for as much of your health care as possible. The amount you are responsible to pay is less than if you go to an out-of-network provider. Sometimes insurance companies pay nothing at all for out-of-network service providers.
- Ask your doctor if they will honor out-of-pocket payment from you at the same rate they are reimbursed by the health care plans they accept. If a doctor nominally charges $200 for a visit, they may only be reimbursed $100 plus your co-pay, so you could save a lot of money, if they say yes.
- Typically, the IRS does not authorize the use of FSA or HSA accounts to pay gym memberships. However, if your doctor writes a pre-

scription for you to enroll in a gym to treat a specific condition, it may be approved by your insurance provider under certain conditions. If a new mattress is prescribed, it is a possibility that your FSA or HSA can be used to pay for it. If massage is deemed a matter of medical necessity, it too can be paid for out of your FSA or HSA account.

- Use your FSA or HSA to pay co-pays for medical appointments, glasses or drugs. Talk to your accountant about any tax benefits that go along with these programs.

- If your employer moves to terminate your job, try to include several months of health insurance coverage in your severance package. Compare your coverage fees for COBRA—which stands for The Consolidated Omnibus Budget Reconciliation Act of 1985—to the coverage fees offered by the exchanges.

- If you are planning to start a new job, determine if there is a waiting period prior to receiving your insurance benefits. A waiting period cannot exceed 90 days. If there is a waiting period, a good option would be to remain on COBRA or purchase a short term private insurance plan to cover the gap.

- Shop around for your medications. Prices can vary widely by pharmacy and there are often coupons available. In addition, if your doctor says it is okay, ask for generic versions of the medications rather than brand names. GoodRx.com is an example of an online site that offers drug comparison-shopping and coupons.

- If you take a medication on a regular basis, ask for ninety-day prescription. This will save you three co-payments. For some medications, and in some plans, a ninety-day prescription is not possible. However, it never hurts to ask.
- If your insurer refuses to cover a procedure, you should always appeal their decision.
- Always check your doctor's bill and compare it to your EOB (Explanation of Benefits) to make sure both are correct.
- Keep a personal copy of your medical records in a place where you can retrieve specific documents before a medical appointment. If your doctor asks you to take a specific test that you've already taken, and you can show the results for that test, you can often avoid the time and expense to repeat it.
- If you are slammed with a large hospital bill that you cannot afford to pay, try negotiating with the hospital. Many have systems and plans in place to schedule smaller payments over time and sometimes you can actually get the price reduced.
- Do the math. This may seem like a no-brainer but add up all the premiums on the higher-level plans plus deductible and compare that information to the higher deductible plans before making a decision on which insurance plan is best for you.

- A visit with a teledoctor may be less expensive than an in-person visit. Patients select tele-medicine for diagnosis of such things as strep throat, acne, anxiety, UTI and other common health problems.
- Take advantage of free wellness visits with your primary care doctor. It's likely your doctor knows a good deal about how insurance works and how you can maximize it.

Switching Plans

If you determine you need to change your insurance plan, you will need to wait a year for open enrollment both in employer and exchange-sponsored programs. There are a few ways to skirt the one-year rule. Here are some tips:

- If you experience a life-changing event, you have thirty days to add to or alter your insurance. Life-changing events include marriage, divorce, domestic violence, flood or other disaster, death, and bankruptcy.
- Keep in mind that insurers cannot deny coverage for a preexisting condition unless it is a grandfathered plan. A grandfathered plan is one purchased on or before March 23, 2010. An insurance company must notify you if you have a grandfathered plan. You can learn more about your options for replacing your

grandfathered plan at this site: https://www.healthcare.gov/health-care-law-protections/grandfathered-plans/

- When you have a baby, provide the baby's social security number and birth certificate to your insurer within thirty days. This will give you the opportunity to make revisions to your plan at that time.

Dr. G's Takeaways

- You need to take a self-inventory to determine your insurance needs.
- If you like your doctor, call and see if he or she is on your plan before you purchase insurance.
- There are numerous different types of plans. Choose the right one for you.
- When you get your policy, be sure to read and understand it.
- Medicare is not free. If you are on Medicare, you can cover co-pays and other expenses out-of-pocket or with supplemental insurance.
- If you feel you will be leaving your job in the near future, use the money in your FSA (Flexible Savings Account), otherwise the money will revert to your employer
- Be aware in most plans, you are almost always required to pay a co-pay even if you have met your deductible.
- If medically possible, leave major procedures until the end of the year when you have met

or almost fully met your deductibles and your total out of pocket expenses.

- Completing a comparison worksheet should give a good overview of what's coming up in the future and how to plan for expenses. You may also decide that you will need to switch to a new plan.
- Plan carefully to maximize your insurance benefits.

PART 3

BEING AND STAYING WELL

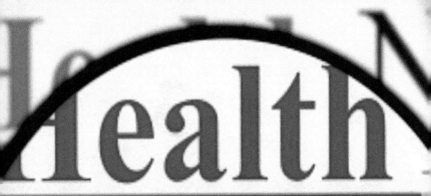

VOL.XI - no.4350

Diabetes

major changes on Earth. We will visit several places of strategic interest and will discuss possible collabora- ns nationally.

Among other th also discuss new on global secu time this me productiv mai

CHAPTER 11

Researching Your Health

> *"Lies run sprints, truth runs marathons."*
> Michael Jackson

As I mentioned in the introduction, part of the impetus for writing this book was the increased number of young patients scaring themselves by trying to self-diagnose through websites like WebMD. They would use the online symptom checker and arrive at a diagnosis based on what they had read, and then make an appointment with me to confirm their diagnosis. Often, they came to my office shaken, believing they had a serious medical condition. After a thorough examination in my office, I was typically able to comfort them with the news that their condition was significantly less serious than what they feared. I would end the appointment with a little guidance about how to research health matters on the Internet. After all, research is part of self-health. I encourage you do research your health online. In this chapter, I am going to show you how to avoid the classic online research mistakes.

Web Research Case # 1: "Would you prescribe this for me?"

Here's a typical scenario: a patient brings me an article or testimonial from a medical professional about a new diet pill that will help them lose weight. They want me to prescribe it for them. The new supplement or medication will come with a series of testimonials and all the right buzz-words—claims that it is "all natural" and has been "used for hundreds of years," etc.

Look at the source of such articles. If the claims being made are found through an online site sponsored by a pharmaceutical company—rather than a peer-reviewed medical journal—then ignore them. A peer-reviewed medical journal is one that focuses on a particular issue of public health and is made available to researchers throughout the world for their input and comment. If the claims *are* from a peer-reviewed medical journal, then look at the study's conclusions and potential side effects. Does the benefit of this supplement, medication or procedure outweigh the risks? Often, it does not, especially if there are alternative methods to achieve a similar health outcome.

Web Research Case # 2: "I think I have cancer."

Another scenario starts with the patient researching common symptoms like "sudden weight loss" or "blood in the stool." Potential diseases like cancer pop up in the results. The patient grows increasingly concerned. They come into my office concerned that they might have terminal cancer. What they haven't taken into account is their medical history—things like a recent trauma, stress, or a history of hemorrhoids or diarrhea or other maladies. When a doctor evaluates a patient's condition, these are among the first contributing factors that he or she will consider.

For this and many reasons, online symptom checkers are usually not that accurate. A study by Harvard Medical School asked 234 doctors to diagnose 45 different clinical descriptions of conditions ranging from canker sores to pulmonary embolism (a dangerous clot in the lung.) They compared the docs' diagnoses to those of a variety of symptom checkers. The checkers identified the likely correct diagnosis just 34 percent of the time, while the doctors' percentage was 72%.

There are any number of medical reasons why a patient might be, for example, experiencing rapid weight loss or have blood in their stool. Stress is a common cause of these symptoms as are diarrheal syndrome or diverticulosis, among others. The internet is a powerful tool, but I do not recommend it for self-diagnosis. What you find online can unnecessarily stress you out. It is far better to consult with your medical practitioner before jumping to conclusions about your health as a result of online research.

Web Research Case # 3: "My friend showed me this article..."

In this scenario a patient requests a prescription for a medication like Adderall to help them focus. They come to my office with a clipping that a friend has printed off the Internet and passed on to them. The friend says she has found Adderall helps her concentrate. The article describes symptoms of adult ADD or ADHD and my patient believes she may be suffering from this condition.

Sponsored journalism—like the articles that appear on WebMD and related sites—are often paid for by pharmaceutical companies. The medical descriptions in these articles invite readers to believe they have a specific condition. They then ask their doctor for a prescription for one of the drugs advertised on the site. It's no wonder that doctors in the U.S. prescribe these kinds of medications at a rate ten times higher than doctors in other countries. It is far better to consult government websites like heart.org or private sites of trusted medical organizations like the Mayo Clinic that do not rely on paid advertisements and sponsorships from drug companies to power their sites.

When a patient comes to me saying he or she believes they have ADD based on what they've read online, the first thing we do is look at the website together in my office. We almost immediately find banner ads next to the article discussing the symptoms of ADD or ADHD for drugs or medicines that will help ADD or ADHD. We then compare the description of ADD or ADHD to the condition's actual DSM V classifications (Diagnostic and Statistical Manual of Mental Disorders, Fifth Edition. Edited by American Psychiatric Association). Invariably, we find a different description.

Web Research Case # 4: "My medication is making me sick!"

I see this scenario frequently: a patient comes into my office believing the medication he has been taking for months or even years is now making him ill. He has read about the medication's side effects online. He has these same symptoms and believes his medication is the reason.

You'd be surprised at the range of symptoms patients blame on their medications. If you've been taking a medication for a period of time and suddenly appear to be suffering from symptoms that you've never experienced before, it's understandable to be alarmed and think they might be side effects from your medication. However, it's important to consider the possibility that these new symptoms might not be related to your medicine at all. If you see a side effect listed for a medication you are taking, research the percentage of the population the side effect impacts as well as when it occurs and in which types of patients.

Finding Reliable Health Websites

We search the Web for many things—information, books, music, electronics, fashion and even dates. Searching for health and medical information is no exceptions. It's easy to get lost in cyberspace once you start. If you go to Google and type in "stomach pains after eating" you will find no less than 1,140,000 sites (in only 38 seconds!) that offer a wide variety of reasons why you may not be feeling good after your evening meal. Here's a random sampling so you can see for yourself:

- Health.com offers "20 Reasons Why Your Stomach Hurts" and includes such things as stress, too much sugarless gum, and ulcers as possible sources of your pain.
- Today.com includes "10 Tummy Troubles You Should Never Ignore" and suggests you may be feeling bad due to thyroid problems, irritable bowel syndrome or even gallstones.
- ReadersDigest.com presents "7 Stomach Pains and What They Mean" and scares you with possible signs of a heart attack, appendicitis or even food poisoning.

It's no wonder that people get confused and even upset when they turn to the Internet to determine what is wrong when they are not feeling well. That's why it's important to evaluate the sites you visit when doing online research about your health. According to the National Center for Complementary and Integrative Health (www. nccih.nih.gov), there are five questions you should ask yourself when you visit and evaluate a health Website for the first time:

- **Who?** Who runs the site? Can you trust them?
- **What?** What does the site say? Do its claims seem too good to be true?
- **When?** When was the information posted or

reviewed? Is it up-to-date?

- **Where?** Where did the information come from? Is it based on scientific research?
- **Why?** Why does the site exist? Is it selling something?

There are many ways to determine if a source of information is respected and credible. One way is to look at the Web address (also called the URL) to see what type of organization is sponsoring the site. Those sponsored by government, educational institutions, or credible professional organizations are more likely to provide unbiased information than commercial sites. You can differentiate sites by looking at the last segment of their URL. If you see .gov, you're looking at a site created by the U.S. government. When you find .edu at the end of a URL, an educational institution has created the site. A site with .org at the end is a professional or non-profit organization. The website that end in .com are commercial and are sponsored by companies—like pharmaceutical companies.

Once you've determined the source of a website's information, here some additional tips and considerations for online health research:

- Oftentimes a website's information has not been updated in months or even years. To check if a website is up to date, scroll down to the bottom of the screen. You should see a sentence that tells you the last time information was posted to the site. If there is no indication or you cannot find a date, assume the information on this site is not current. Poor design, broken links and technical flaws on a site should also give you pause.

- Credible sites will always have links to their sources, additional information, quotes from experts, etc. If you don't see these present on a site, do not trust the information there.
- If something "sounds too good to be true," trust your instincts—it probably is. Be especially wary of those who promise a "miracle cure."
- Be particularly wary of sites that feature banner ads for the latest pharmaceutical products. The content on these sites has an agenda. The goal is to get you to ask for a prescription or purchase an over-the-counter drug based on what you learn there.
- Beware of sites that overuse the "celebrity effect." While the death of a celebrity from a particular illness often raises public awareness to the disease in question and can lead to beneficial discussions about treatment options, remember that each one of us is different. How a disease or condition manifests and progresses varies from one person to the next. If you have a concern, consult your doctor. They know you and your unique medical history.

- Verify health claims that are based on personal testimony through multiple credible sources. Online support groups, forums or blogs are a great way to share experiences and information. However, they should not be used for diagnosis.
- Assess the strength of health claims presented online. For example, a health claim based on one small study is not as strong as a health claim based on the findings of multiple large-scale studies.
- To get to the most precise information quickly, be specific in your online searches. If you're looking for information about depression during the holidays, don't just type the phrase "depression and the holidays." Instead, put an exact question into quotations as a search term, such as "Why do people get depressed around the holidays?" You are more likely to find the exact information you are looking for in the top ten or twenty search results that pop up.

Some Reliable Sites on the Internet

Here are some sites I recommend that can be trusted when researching health and medical information online:

Mayo Clinic

www.mayoclinic.org/
This is one of my all-time favorite websites. The database in the lifestyle section is exhaustive and authoritative. You can also research both symptoms and diagnoses. One goal of the site is to increase referrals to the Mayo Clinic, which I find an acceptable objective as it doesn't seem to influence the credibility of the scientifically document information that is shared on the site.

Medline Plus

www.medlineplus.gov
This site is an amazing clearinghouse of credible information, all of which is public domain. There is also an exhaustive list of natural substances and supplements available on the site. The information is divided into three sections:

- health topics—medical conditions, therapies and wellness
- drugs and supplements
- videos and tools

It is truly an amazing and helpful database. MedlinePlus is updated daily and there is no advertising on the site. Additionally, MedlinePlus does not endorse any company or product.

NIH Senior Health

www.nia.nih.gov/health
The site created by the National Institutes of Health has a tremendous amount of information for the elderly and the health-related issues specific to this age group.

Healthfinder

www.Healthfinder.gov
This is the Grand Central Station of sites to help you find a wide range of health topics that are covered by more than a thousand government and nonprofit organizations.

Sharing Web Research with Your Doctor

There is nothing wrong with using the Internet to research information to help you manage your health and wellness. However, it is important to understand that online research should never replace a conversation with your doctor. If you have questions or concerns about a particular health issue, make an appointment. If an online article concerns you, it's a good idea to print them out and bring it to your appointment.

Dr. G's Takeaways

- Understand the type of site your viewing during your online research—is the site a .gov, .org or a .com?
- Beware of the "celebrity effect" and outrageous claims.
- Seek out reliable online resources that are not sponsorship-driven.
- Make sure claims are from peer-reviewed medical journals.
- Beware of the health sites that have a lot of banner ads.
- Bring in the clippings from your internet research to discuss with your doctor openly to see what he or she thinks of the information.

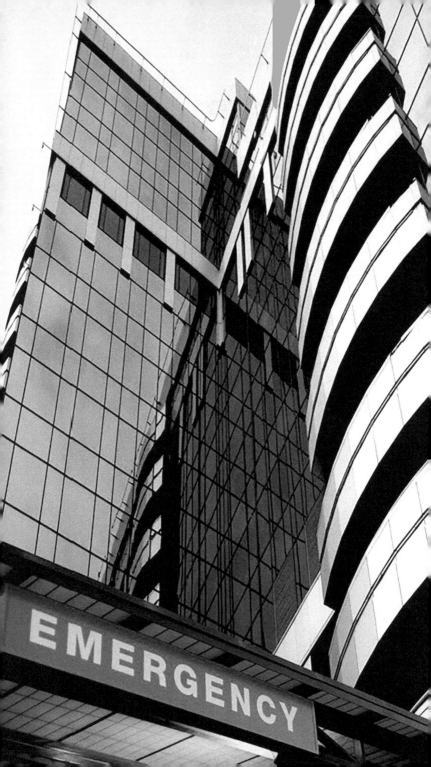

CHAPTER 12

Managing Medical Emergencies

> *"Stay calm inside. You'll see the outside
> storms of life—even the most powerful
> ones—will turn to soft winds."*
>
> *Mehmet Murat IIdan, Turkish writer*

I once produced radio show called "Life in the Balance," in which I interviewed paramedics about their experiences in the field. I was surprised to learn that in car crashes, the intoxicated driver often walks away without a scratch. Sadly, the person in the other car would sustain injuries or be killed. As he or she remains physically relaxed during the crash, the drunk driver wouldn't go into shock. Paramedics mentioned that the intoxicated driver would "bounce" on impact and hence not sustain any injuries. In contrast, the alert driver in the other car would mentally and physically tense up and hold onto the steering wheel so tight that on impact sometimes their wrists would snap. What a sad realization. We can, however, learn from this. The takeaway is that if you if remain mentally and physically calm in emergencies, you stand a better chance.

Preparing for Medical Emergencies

No one ever wakes up and declares, "Today I will have a medical emergency!" If they did, they might be better prepared for what lies ahead. But the reality is, we take life for granted and always assume that "everything will be just fine." Then a car runs a red light and hits you, or you don't pay attention while walking down the stairs and you fall. Any number of obstacles and hazards are placed in our way each day. How well you are prepared will determine your outcome. For example, if you are a strong defensive driver then your chances of being in a car crash are less than those of the person who doesn't really pay attention to the cars around them on the road. And if you hold the handrails with both hands while walking down the stairs (instead of texting or looking at your smartphone!) you stand a better chance of not falling down.

Your first-aid kit

The Boys Scouts have a great motto: "Be Prepared." That's all you need to remember and know. Be prepared. The first rule of being prepared is to be ready for any medical emergency. You can accomplish this goal by having a good first aid kit on hand. You can purchase one from your local pharmacy or even the supermarket. And a quick search online will give you plenty of options to choose from.

You also need to have a good first aid kit in your car. But don't do what most people do and purchase one, put it in the trunk, console or glove compartment, and never look at it again until you need it. Some items in the kit will expire, and it never hurts to check to see if everything looks like it's in good shape at least once a year or more often.

Some people prefer to create their own kit, which is also a good idea. Plastic boxes or containers can be filled with the same supplies purchased at Walgreens, Rite-Aid, etc. According to the American Red Cross, the following items should be included in any standard First Aid Kit:

2 absorbent compress dressings (5 x 9 inches)
25 adhesive bandages (assorted sizes)
1 adhesive cloth tape (10 yards x 1 inch)
5 antibiotic ointment packets (approximately 1 gram)
5 antiseptic wipe packets
2 packets of aspirin (81 mg each)
1 blanket (space blanket)

1 breathing barrier (with one-way valve)
1 instant cold compress
2 pair of nonlatex gloves (size: large)
2 hydrocortisone ointment packets (approximately 1 gram each)
Scissors
1 roller bandage (3 inches wide)
1 roller bandage (4 inches wide)
5 sterile gauze pads (3 x 3 inches)
5 sterile gauze pads (4 x 4 inches)
Oral thermometer (non-mercury/nonglass)
2 triangular bandages
Tweezers
First aid instruction booklet

You should also include the names and contact information of your doctors, you and anyone in your family in the first aid kit and in the glove box of your car.

Home and Office Emergency Plan

No matter where you are employed, you should be aware of the location of the first aid kits and know how to help someone should an emergency take place. Most large companies will have first aid kits on hand as well as an automated external defibrillator (AED). If your employer does not, then you should suggest they do.

Knowing what to do should an emergency occur at home or at the office is a good idea. When you're in school, you are taught about fire prevention safety tips, and families are encouraged to create a plan of escape *before* it is necessary. The time to think about what to do and where to go is not in the middle of an emergency.

Be sure you know the location of the nearest emergency room or urgent care facility, but at the same time, understand what your insurance company will cover. If it's a matter of life or death, get the life-saving measures you or someone else needs first and worry about the insurance company later. However, if it is not a serious life or death situation, understanding what your insurance will cover and *where* it will cover treatment is good to know ahead of time. If you are not sure, then check with your insurance provider. And when you are going on vacation or traveling for work, it's a good idea to research local hospitals, etc. before you leave home.

Your Medical History on Your Person

Having a complete list of medications, complications, and any other important information with you at all times will make things much easier in the event you find yourself in an emergency situation.

Knowing your medical history makes it much easier for an emergency room doctor to treat you, which is why I highly recommend keeping your medical history on your person at all times. Whether you have a paper file, or keep an electronic record on your smartphone, it will save time, and also in many cases, costs. When you are doubled over in pain, the last thing you want is to play twenty questions with an emergency room person who really needs that important information.

The Office of the Surgeon General offers a tool called My Family Health Portrait that allows you to enter, print, and update your family health history. You can find it at https://familyhistory.hhs.gov/FHH/html/index.html

The American Medical Association also provides medical history tools, including questionnaires and forms for collecting medical information. You can find it at

https://www.ama-assn.org/delivering-care/collecting-family-history

Emergency 101: When You Need to Call 911

There will be times in your life when you experience a real emergency. You might witness a car crash and dial 911, or someone in the supermarket collapses and stops breathing. These are examples of situations when calling the 911 operating system is the appropriate course of action. Each year, however, thousands of calls are made to 911 operators that are not for true emergencies. Be sure it really is an emergency before casually calling 911.

It isn't unusual for people to become upset in an emergency situation, but when you call 911 stay calm and think logically; help will be on the way faster than if you sob and cry into the phone and no one can understand what you're saying. When an emergency occurs, it is common for your body to quickly move into the "fight or flight" mode, which means your body will immediately start producing the stress hormone cortisol that goes directly to your brain. If you're not careful, your thought processing ability will soon slow down and even become slightly impaired. Take a deep breath, organize your thoughts, and calmly state what the emergency is, the location, and the condition of the parties who need medical help, and a call-back number. If you know the medical history of the people involved, such as medical conditions, medications, allergies and past surgeries, be prepared to share it with the emergency personnel as this will make their jobs easier.

Minute Clinic, Urgent Care Center, or Emergency Room?

No one can predict when they will wake up with extreme stomach pain, or if they will fall in the parking lot of the supermarket. And if you have children, you know that one minute they may be laughing and playing and the next minute be suffering from an ear-ache that is driving them (and you) crazy. In the old days, you could call the family doctor, or they would even visit your home. Then emergency rooms started opening in hospitals all across the country, and before long, the ER was the place to go if you ran into trouble.

Although the first urgent care center opened in 1970, it wasn't until about fifteen years ago or so that they started also appearing in shopping centers and strip malls. Some are only open during daytime hours, while others are open until late in the evening. A great number of them are now operating twenty-four hours a day. Visit any large city and you will probably find a few urgent care centers, some within blocks of each other.

It can often be difficult to decide whether you should go to the emergency room or simply try out an urgent care center. Oftentimes the wait is considerably shorter at the urgent care centers, but keep in mind they are limited in how they can treat certain medical emergencies. The rule of thumb is "urgent care is not emergency care." So, if what you are experiencing is a life-threatening emergency, go to the emergency room. If you have a minor illness, fever, sore throat, etc., and your primary care physician is unavailable, then an urgent care center will be fine.

Urgent care centers, unlike minute clinics in drugstores are equipped to treat cuts, burns, strains, sprains, bites and any number of medical problems. You should always check with your health insurance provider ahead of time though, to make sure what treatments they will cover. Research online or call your neighborhood immediate care and urgent care centers to see what they can handle in order to get a better sense of where to go when you have health issues.

If you are, in doubt about the severity the medical situation, head to the nearest emergency room facility. They are equipped to handle any type of medical emergency or condition and are staffed with doctors, nurses and other medical staff to assist those in need.

Navigating Emergency Facilities

When you are taken by an ambulance to an emergency room at the hospital there is a special entrance reserved for what may be life-threatening conditions: heart attacks, strokes, gunshot wounds, etc. If you walk into the emergency room, or have someone bring you, and it does not appear that you need immediate medical attention to stay alive, an ER staff person will take your information, and a practitioner will provide an initial examination and then determine when you will be treated. This occurs after a basic triage process to determine that you're able to wait.

In the emergency room, if you need immediate medical attention, (for example, you cut your hand and it won't stop bleeding), they will quickly assess the situation and put you in what is known as the "fast track." You will receive those much-needed stitches, so the bleeding will stop. However, if you visit the emergency room with severe stomach pains, the medical personnel will need to do some additional evaluations to determine what the problem might be.

A blood test will let the practitioner know if what you are experiencing is an appendicitis attack or just a regular stomach ache. Xrays and other medical tests will take a while to complete and review the results, and a specialist may even need to be called in for a consultation. In either case, you will be stabilized, and if need be, placed in a waiting area until someone can see you.

If your visit to the emergency room is for something minor, like a sore throat or an upset stomach—as opposed to a dire medical situation in which you are in danger of bleeding to death—your visit will most likely last for three or more hours, depending upon the size of the ER, how busy it is at the time, and the number of medical personnel on staff.

After being treated in ER, and assuming you are not being admitted into the hospital, you will receive your discharge papers. These will include vital information about your condition, the treatment that was provided, any medications that were received, and most importantly, instructions on how and when to follow up with your primary care doctor. DO NOT ignore those instructions! If there is something on the form that you do not agree with, or understand, by all means ask questions and get clarification.

Sadly, only a small percentage of people who have visited an emergency room or urgent care center ever bother to follow up with their primary care doctor. They automatically assume that since they were not admitted as a patient, were discharged and possibly given some medications, that all is right with their world. But that is not true. If you look carefully at the discharge or treatment papers that you are given when you leave the ER or urgent care facility, it will ALWAYS tell you to "follow up with your primary care physician."

When you make an appointment to see your doctor after your ER visit, be sure to bring all of the paperwork with you. Do not assume that your doctor has received any or all of the information that was provided. And remember, you need to understand the emergency evaluation summary and discharge papers that were given to you. Ask questions if you don't understand something. No one is going to yell or be mad at you, trust me. The more informed you are, the better!

If you were given any medications or a prescription for medications, be sure to let your doctor know you are taking them. Also check with your pharmacist to make sure that any medications you were prescribed will not have adverse reactions to any existing ones you are already taking.

Dr. G's Takeaways

- It's important during an emergency to remain calm and relay your story carefully.
- When speaking to the 911 operator, relate the nature of the emergency, the name of the people involved (if known), your location, the condition of the injured person as well as your callback number.

- All emergencies cannot be avoided but practicing good prevention (like being a defensive driver) is the best way to avoid emergencies.
- A first-aid kit should close at hand at all times—in your home, place of work and car.
- Keep your medical history on your person, which at the very least should include a list of diagnoses, medicines and allergies to medicines.
- Study on the web or call and ask questions of your neighborhood immediate care and urgent care centers to see what they can handle to have a better sense of where to go when you have a health issue.
- There are some circumstances where fast track injuries like stitches take place in other parts of the emergency room, and then there are more involved evaluations that require blood tests, or xrays consultations with other specialists.
- It's important to always follow up with your primary care doctor after an emergency room visit and bring your discharge summary with your diagnoses and medications.
- A staycation can be as beneficial as a vacation, but you have to get in the right mindset to believe that you are a vacation at home.
- A transformative vacation works because you're using the insights that you gained during your vacation and applying them to your life at home.

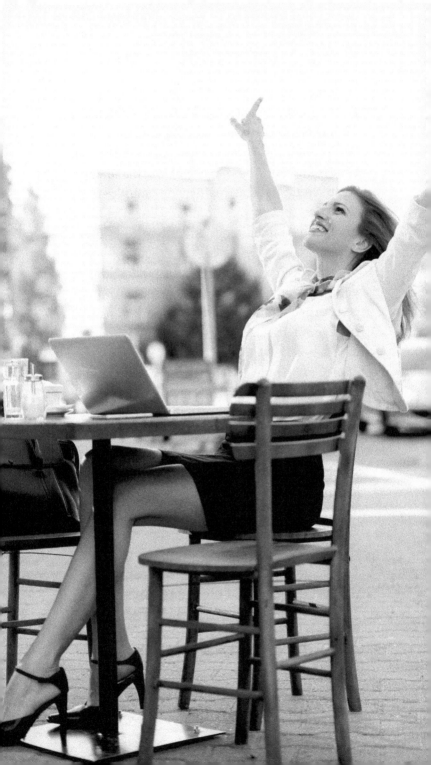

CHAPTER 13

Rewarding Yourself the Healthy Way

> *"The reward of a thing well done is to have done it."*
>
> Ralph Waldo Emerson

" I apologize but we are all out of confetti!" I commonly joke and simultaneously congratulate my patients when they come for an office visit and report that they have lost the first ten pounds toward their weight goal or have a reached another health milestone that they established. I very much enjoy the role of being a witness to the health progress of others. whether it be smoking cessation, achieving optimal blood sugar levels in my diabetics, or weight loss in my overweight patients.

Learn to celebrate your achievements and milestones on the way to self-health. In this chapter,

I will discuss how to create healthy and motivating rewards for yourself. I will introduce you to intertwining methods of self-reflection, self-motivation, self-congratulation and partnering with a health buddy to celebrate your accomplishments. Cheat days, "staycations" and transformational vacations all play a vital role in keeping you healthy, happy and fit in both body and mind. Here's how to successfully navigate the terrain of saluting yourself for a job well done.

Reward Yourself When You Achieve Your Health Goals

It is always wonderful to receive acknowledgement for a big personal accomplishment like lowering your cholesterol. We need to stop and take time to applaud ourselves. But this does not necessarily mean eating an entire cake, guzzling an entire bottle of champagne, or going on a five-hour shopping binge. What it means is enjoying a welcome respite, celebrating in your own way and evaluating next steps.

Solid relationships and positive reinforcement can work wonders when trying to motivate yourself to make healthy lifestyle changes. While Janis did not experience much difficulty in reducing the salt in her diet, many people discover it is not as easy as it seems to give up pizza, cake, smoking or binge-watching the latest television miniseries for four hours a day from your sofa (sometimes while consuming all of the aforementioned). A friendly pat on the back, or a hearty "Job well done!" goes a long way for someone who has put forth the effort to kick unhealthy habits to the curb.

My patient Janis told me she wanted to take steps to lower her blood pressure. She began with the easiest step, reducing the amount of salt in her diet. She then began walking three or four times a week. Finally, she added meditation to combat her stress and calm her mind. Her husband was her health buddy. Not only did he keep her on track, he joined her on her walks. When Janis successfully brought her blood pressure down to the 120s over 80s range, she celebrated by treating herself to dinner out with her health buddy.

It is important that we reward ourselves as we reach our goals, but little rewards to celebrate milestones along the way are also important. If your goal is to lose 30 pounds, reflecting and cheering each of the 10 pounds you lose along the way is its own accomplishment and should be duly recognized. Once you reach each goalpost on your way to success, take a step back and notice if your behavior has changed in any way. Determine how you can create a healthy new habit instead of going back to negative behaviors and thus undermining your efforts. In other words, it's important to reflect on what you did right when you achieve your health goal, so you can learn from this and perhaps apply these actions to other health and life goals you might have.

Health Breaks and Cheat Days

As I discussed earlier, not all stress is bad. Stress can trigger great spurts of energy and creativity, but it can also trigger anxiety, depression, and sleeplessness. Even people who thrive on stress need an occasional break. If you are burning the candle at both ends, you should occasionally schedule a cheat day or a mental health day to rejuvenate.

I know when I'm getting a little too stressed-out—or "crispy," as I like to call it. If I am having trouble remembering names or just not as sharp as I should be, I try to step back and recharge. Pay attention to when you feel overwhelmed, stressed and not functioning at one hundred percent. That's when it's time to take a break—even if it's just for one cheat day or mental health day.

If you are planning your mental health day in advance, it is a good idea to think about why you need it. Are you stressed about money? Are you dissatisfied with your job? Your life? The mundane aspects of the everyday grind? If you can pinpoint the cause of your stress, you can schedule the right kind of relaxation and then—rejuvenated after your break—you can tackle the issue that is making you stressed. If you're feeling hemmed in? Opt for a change of scenery by taking a drive or checking into a hotel for the day and ordering room service. Feeling tense about work? Have a massage. Think about ways to improve your situation and write them down. If you are worried, meditate, do yoga or just veg on your sofa. Bored and not challenged? Attend a lecture or concert or watch a DIY video on YouTube.

You should also reward yourself for being disciplined and sticking to your self-health plan. Take a day off from your diet or exercise plan. For one day, treat yourself. This doesn't mean you can go hog-wild; it means you can take a break from grilled chicken breasts, kale salad and six-mile run for one day. Everyone suffers from food and exercise boredom. Perhaps on your cheat day, you enjoy a small dessert, add a special sauce to your chicken, fix a "forbidden" side dish for dinner and take a walk instead of run. There is evidence that an occasional cheat day can even assist your weight loss program by helping your body maintain energy levels needed to continue dieting and exercising. A young patient of mine named Lisbeth had shed twelve pounds on her way to losing a total of twenty-five pounds. Since she'd hit the halfway mark, she decided to treat herself to a special book.

She took the day off from work to read it. Mental health and cheat days don't have to be extravagant or pricey, they just need to be fun and stress free.

Taking Time Away

A recent study by Gallup revealed that adults who are employed full time report work an average of forty-seven hours per week. This equates to nearly six days a week. And nearly four in ten workers report logging more than fifty hours of work each week. Clearly, America's behavior and attitudes toward work-life balance are, well, not in balance. I see how this impacts my patients all the time. Erik, who is only 32 years old, came to see me for a wellness check and told me that he had begun working out during lunch in an effort build energy and stamina. "That's great," I told him. "You should reward yourself. Get away somewhere." Erik confessed he rarely vacationed and did not even take time off for public holidays. I asked him if his employer was compensating him for all of his extra hard work. The answer was "no." To Erik, and the many people like Erik, I explain, "Refusing to take a break is holding you back."

Project: Time Off is a national movement to share the value of taking time off. This coalition of organizations wants to change America's behavior and attitudes about work-life balance. On average, Project: Time Off found that employees who did not take a break "donated" $604 back to their employers. Even more disappointing, Project: Time Off discovered that thirty-eight percent of employees said they want to be seen as a work martyr by their boss. Project: Time Off's website states: "What those nearly four-in-ten employees do not understand is that work martyrdom not only does not help them advance in their careers; it may be hurting them."

Despite the growing body of evidence that too much work is not good for our productivity or health, we continue working too many hours, nonstop for long periods of time. If you fall into this group, I first challenge you to figure out your reason for doing this. Second, I challenge you to try a vacation and see if it actually improves your productivity and well-being.

Indulge in a "staycation"

If you can't afford the time or money to take a full-blown vacation, consider a "staycation"—when you stay home, but pretend you're on vacation and do everything that you would do on that vacations. They are good for stress reduction, improved productivity, gaining a new outlook on life, controlling heart disease and managing your relationships. There are advantages, of course, to going away on a real vacation, however, if planned correctly, a staycation can also make you feel relaxed and rejuvenated.

A staycation is designed to help you forget about work and responsibilities for a healthy period of time—anywhere from one full day, to a couple days or an entire week or more. Perhaps you visit the sites in your city that you've never visited or do something creative giving your staycation a theme. For example, you could take three days off and do a tour of the Italian provinces. Order posters in advance from your favorite Italian cities—Venice, Naples, Florence, and Rome, for example. Put the posters up in your home. Then prepare culinary delights from each city: Neapolitan pizza on Friday, Chicken Florentine on Saturday, and Sicilian shrimp pasta on Sunday. Maybe one night, you have a dinner party in your new Italian villa and greet your guests the Italian way by kissing them on each side of the cheek. The important thing is to make it fun and stress-free. Here are some tips for setting up a staycation:

- Set a date.
- Plan your theme, "A weekend in Paris", "A week cruise on the Pacific."
- Decide who will be joining you.
- Set a budget.
- Arrange for your landlines to be turned off
- Stop delivery of your paper.

- Turn on "the away from" message on your work email
- Disconnect from social media on your computer and on your phone.
- If you are not planning to "take" your children on your staycation, arrange for a sitter or parent or friend to care for them. You can arrange a share plan with a friend, where you will watch their kids.
- If your kids are "coming" with you on your staycation, plan family-friendly outings
- If you care for older adults look into respite or ask a sibling or friend to help you out for a short period of time.
- Shop for all necessary food before your vacation and stock your refrigerator or arrange for supermarket delivery.
- Clean your house before you "embark."
- If the weather is nice, try to do things outdoors.
- Try to learn something new. Visit a museum you wanted to see. Go to movies.
- Do not be tempted to check your work email.
- Stay away from household projects.
- Add turn down service. Put a chocolate on your pillow and a flower by your bedside.
- Have a massage, take a yoga class. Explore your neighborhood. Do something new.
- Book a hotel room nearby if you like. The rates may be better during a weekday.
- Turn off all thoughts of housekeeping. No laundry, dusting or vacuuming.

You will "return" from your staycation renewed, refreshed, and recharged.

Transformative vacations

Transformative vacations are growing in popularity. They require an investment of time and money, which may put them out of reach for some. A transformative vacation is designed to shift your perspective or give you time to learn something new. When you return, you put your newfound perspective and knowledge into action in your day-to-day life. A truly transformative vacation requires a week or more for an optimal experience.

Here are some suggestions for how to create a fulfilling transformational vacation. Start by making a list what you want to change in life—maybe it's your overall mindset or your maybe your goal is to quit smoking—or something you'd like to learn—how to surf or how to paint, scuba dive or cook Italian food. While you can take a transformative vacation near home, a new setting is preferred. It's part of the transformative experience. Where have you always wanted to visit? What culture intrigues you? What languages would you like to learn? If your ultimate goal is personal transformation, make time on your vacation to contemplate the changes you want to see in your life and why you want to make those changes. Take time to read, write and think about these changes. You'll be amazed by

Dr. G's Takeaways

- Don't work too much. Take a break. It is critical to productivity and well-being.
- Reward yourself for reaching goals.
- Enjoy an occasional cheat day.
- Plan a staycation or transformative vacation for rejuvenation.

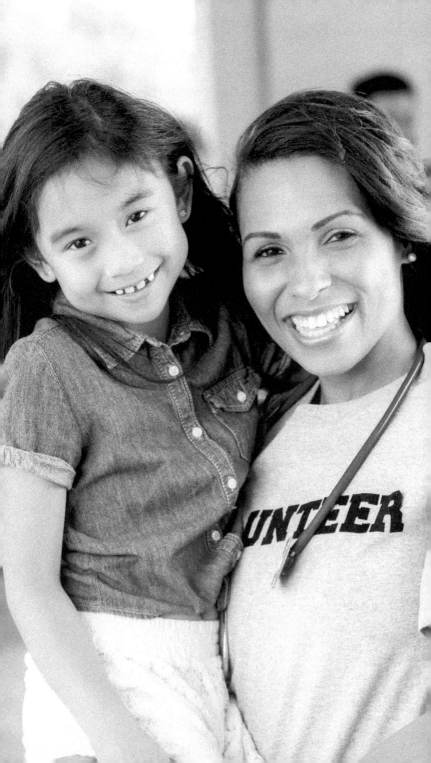

CHAPTER 14

Paying It Forward

> *"I alone cannot change the world, but I can cast a stone across the waters to create many ripples."*
>
> Mother Teresa

"See one, do one, teach one." This is something I first learned from one of my interns when I was a medical student. Since then, I've heard it many times in the medical community. This customarily refers to learning some procedure—perhaps simple suturing or putting a breathing tube down someone—practicing that procedure until you master it, and then demonstrating the skill to others. In medicine, it is how wisdom is passed from skilled clinicians to the next generation of doctors.

We can bring this same practice into self-health. Learn something, practice it and pass it on to others. Let's say you've struggled with anxiety and you've overcome it with through a variety of learned skills and holistic practices—deep breathing, relaxation, progressive muscle relaxation. The next time you meet someone struggling with anxiety, you have an opportunity to pay it forward. You can share what you've learned and help improve someone else's life. Did you know that every time you teach someone else, it reinforces the knowledge you have? So not only will you be helping another human being, you'll be retaining the skills you have learned.

I'm not telling you anything you don't already know, but I would like to encourage you to do this not only to make the world a better place, but for the health benefits. As Saint Francis of Assis famously said, "it is in giving that we receive." There is a now is a growing body of research to support the idea that giving to others actually improves well-being and overall health. Chemicals in our brain like dopamine, serotonin and oxytocin—sometimes called the "Happiness Trifecta"—are triggered by acts of giving. Paying it forward is a win-win situation. You help others and you help yourself. There are a number of ways you can pay it forward on both a small and large scale. Here are some ideas:

Share your story

It takes courage to open up to others about challenges we've faced an overcome. If you're ready, and you can help someone who is struggling, consider sharing your story with them. There may be uncomfortable moments. However, consider the idea that you could change someone's life with your story.

Connect others with resources

If you're comfortable sharing your story, the natural next step is to start sharing the resources that helped you. This is how many bloggers, thought leaders and community organizers got their start. There are so many ways to share in today's mobile, social world. You can start a blog, visit chat rooms on select topics, give a talk at your local library, start a YouTube channel, to name just a few. Sites like Reddit have places called subreddits where a whole community of people with similar medical concerns could converse about all kinds of popular issues. You can find a list of a lot of these subreddits in r/Health. Contributing to the online conversation allows you to share with others while continuing to learn from the community. Everyone benefits.

Strengthen your community

Is there something you could do to better the life of a family member, neighbor or someone in your community? Leo Tolstoy, one of the greatest writers of all time, once said, *"The sole meaning of life is to serve humanity."* Don't be afraid to serve your community. We are all healthier when we live in healthy families, neighborhoods and communities. Consider how you can get involved and give back. This can be as simple as being a role model in your family to volunteering at a local soup kitchen or nursing home to starting a community garden. Get creative and think about how the unique knowledge you gained on your self-health journey could strengthen people and organizations in your community.

Become an advocate

Should you choose to give back on a larger scale, you may want to look into national organizations that can support your efforts. For mental health issues, for example, there is The National Alliance on Mental Illness (NAMI), which encourages people to submit stories to empower those living with mental illnesses through creative means like prose, storytelling, songs, and videos. If you want to advocate for more fitness in America, IDEAfit is comprised of about 250,000 fitness professionals who want to help others become more fit. An organization called Partners in Health has a mission to help build health systems and provide care for countries experiencing poverty. On the food and nutrition front, there are national groups like Feeding America and the more global group Oxfam America. Both groups deal with issues such as poverty, social impact, hunger, and health. Should you have the time and passion, you might be able to find a position at one or more of these organizations where you could contribute or volunteer more actively.

Dr. G's Takeaways

- When you are comfortable, start sharing your health story and the resources that helped you.
- Consider ways to give back to your family, neighbors and community.
- If you're ready to give back on a larger scale, seek out national organizations that might be able to support you.
- Remember, giving back is a win-win situation—not only do can you help others, you may actually see some health benefits yourself.

Conclusion

T hank you for the opportunity to share my philosophy of self-health with you. Putting together this book has been an amazing, reflective journey. Getting my twenty years of experience—with all the joys and struggles of patient care—down on paper has been cathartic. I love what I do, and the process of writing this book has made me a better doctor.

Remember, self-health starts with an honest conversation with yourself. Are you truly healthy? Pretty much everyone on the planet has room for improvement in their health and well-being. Confront the roadblocks that keep you from achieving your health goals—especially fear, stress and loneliness. Overcome these roadblocks with hope, hardiness and support. Be aware of your biases and open to different types of solutions. Don't go it alone. Reach out and find a health buddy who can help you out on your path to better health.

Self-health means taking responsibility for your health. Here are some parting tips—the main pearls that are imparted in the book. Do your homework and understand best practices for researching your symptoms online. Visit reliable sites and follow up with your health-care provider for definitive diagnosis and treatment. Don't be afraid to reach out when you're in over your head. When you need to enter the health care system, be prepared. Understand which systems and personnel with whom you need to interact. Develop long-term, simpatico relationships with your health care providers. Invest the necessary time to completely understand your insurance policy and develop an annual health budget. Your primary care doctor can help with prior authorizations and some of the other headaches associated with insurance.

All of the above are important aspect of your self-health plan. Undertaking these practices will result in many benefits for your health and well-being throughout your life. This is what I wish for you. To your health!

~ Dr. Dominic Gaziano

About the Author

Dominic Gaziano, M.D—known as Dr. G. to his patients—is a practicing adult primary care physician and director of the Body and Mind Medical Center in Chicago. He was the director of the integrative medicine department at Advocate Illinois Masonic Hospital, overseeing programs integrating both western and eastern health practitioners. Trained in western medicine and having interacted with many holistic practitioners, Dr. G. offers the best research-based therapeutic strategies from both eastern and western perspectives.

For more than two decades, Dr. G. has been a relentless advocate for his lower and middle income inner-city patients, helping them find ways to take care of themselves—often despite difficult insurance scenarios and/or limited access to the larger health care system.

Dr. G is one of seven members of his family that have taken the Hippocratic Oath. He draws from his upbringing in a gregarious Italian family, as inspiration for the talk therapy he uses with his patients to help them deal with stress and psycho-social issues. He believes spending time with his patients and talking things out leads to better health-care outcomes with fewer drug prescriptions and less medical intervention. As an advocate of preventative medicine, he encourages his patients to practice self-health in order to lead happy and healthier lives

Well Now! is based on Dr. Gaziano's many years of listening and reflecting upon his thousands of patient encounters in a variety of health-care settings—as outpatients, in hospitals, and in physical rehab settings, among others.

Index

A

E

J – K

O

P – Q

R

CPSIA information can be obtained
at www.ICGtesting.com
Printed in the USA
LVHW081629040219
606328LV00031B/1568/P